THE CHRISTIAN HEALTH MANUAL

THE CHRISTIAN HEALTH MANUAL

Dr Robert Peprah-Gyamfi

Published by THANK YOU JESUS BOOKS

For information, please contact:
THANK YOU JESUS BOOKS
P.O. BOX 8505
LOUGHBOROUGH
LE11 9BZ
UK
www.thankyoujesusbooks.com
ISBN: 978-0-9564734-6-2

All scripture references are from the King James Version

Cover illustration and design by Kristine Cotterman (www.exodusdesign.com).

To Christian Missionary Doctors—past, present and future.

Is any sick among you? let him call for the elders of the church; and let them pray over him, anointing him with oil in the name of the Lord: And the prayer of faith shall save the sick, and the Lord shall raise him up; and if he have committed sins, they shall be forgiven him.

James 5 14 & 15

And lest I should be exalted above measure through the abundance of the revelations, there was given to me a thorn in the flesh, the messenger of Satan to buffet me, lest I should be exalted above measure.
For this thing I besought the Lord thrice, that it might depart from me. And he said unto me, My grace is sufficient for thee: for my strength is made perfect in weakness. Most gladly therefore will I rather glory in my infirmities, that the power of Christ may rest upon me.

2 Corinthians 12: 7-9

Also by Robert Peprah-Gyamfi

1) **Seeing God Through the Human Body:**
   A Doctor's Meditation on the Human Miracle
   Anomalos Publishing, 2009. ISBN: 978-0981764399

2) **Three Cheers for Ghana!**
   IUniverse, 2008. ISBN: 0-595-48523-5

3) **Be Encouraged in Jesus**
   Xulon Press, 2007. ISBN: 0-595-32298-0

4) **A Letter to My Dying Mother**
   Surviving in the West
   iUniverse, 2005. ISBN: 0-595-34794-0

5) **The Call that Changed my Life**
   Thank You Jesus Books, 2010. ISBN: 978-0-9564734-1-7

6) **Doctor Jesus, the Doctor who knows no bounds**
   Thank You Jesus Books, 2010. ISBN: 987-0-9564734-0-0

7) **The Christian Soldier's Battle Cry**
   Thank You Jesus Books, 2010. ISBN: 987-0-9564734-2-4

8) **Growing Up in a Small African Village**
   Perseverance Books, 2010. ISBN: 978-0-9564734-3-1

9) **Growing up in a Small African Village, An Abridged Edition**
   Perseverance Books, 2010. ISBN: 978-0-9564734-4-8

10) **Growing Up in a Little African Village (Children's Edition)**
   Perseverance Books, 2010. ISBN: 978-0-9564734-5-5

TABLE OF CONTENTS

∽

Acknowledgements

My heartfelt thanks go to God Almighty, Creator of heaven and earth, for imparting the wisdom needed to write this book. Rita, my wife, together with our children Karen, David, and Jonathan, also deserve my thanks and appreciation for their support and encouragement, which enabled me to persevere to the successful conclusion of this work. I am also grateful to Dr Charles Muller of Diadembooks.com for carrying out the editorial work and for writing the foreword.

FOREWORD

T his is a health education manual with a difference! First, it is clearly
written, in a friendly and easy to follow manner that will make it
invaluable for the layman who does not have a full understanding of how
the human body functions, to come to grips with the essential causes of
diseases and medical cures. The writer, himself a medical doctor, often
writes from the perspective of his own early background in a rural village
in Ghana, and, indeed, for anyone growing up in an African context, this
book will be a wonderful guide to better health. The analogies the writer
uses make it so much clearer for the reader to grasp the functions of the
body, as when he compares the make-up of the genes and DNA to a football
team! Then again, this book is unique in so far as it is addressed largely to
the Christian reader. The writer's explanation of the nature of disease makes
abundant sense, tracing, as he does, its origin to the fall of man in Eden,
where the Creator made everything perfect and saw that "all was good". His
explanation of cancer, and the parallel he draws with sin, where uncontrolled
cell division equates with uncontrolled human behaviour that "is good for
nothing", is brilliant if not inspired! From a medical and Christian point of
view this book will advocate a lifestyle that will best serve the reader to
prevent disease, for prevention is always better than cure! And where a cure
is needed, the right mental attitude, not forgetting the unlimited power of
prayer, is probably the most important resource.

The manual might be said to be the culmination, not only of the writer's
medical training and experience as a doctor, but of a series of books he has
already penned, all from the perspective of a Christian doctor. Recently he
was interviewed in the London studios of Revelation TV about his books,

which testify to the power of prayer, the power of the Holy Spirit through Faith. In his book *Doctor Jesus: The Doctor who Knows no Bounds*, he demonstrates our Lord's miraculous power of healing, where damaged tissue and bone, even putrefying tissue, is healed instantly, in a matter of seconds—in the "twinkling of an eye". This, in effect, is the power of the resurrection, where damaged or dead tissue or bone is regenerated in an instant in the hands of the Creator, the original designer of the human body. Such healing that we perceive as miraculous still takes place today, and in his new book Dr Peprah-Gyamfi is certainly mindful of this, though at the same time he exhorts the patient to follow his or her doctor's prescriptions and recommended treatment, and in the course of prayer, perhaps occasionally cease the medication to see if the illness has indeed been cured by divine intervention, then resume the doctor's orders if this has not been the case. If a miraculous cure has not taken place, then the Lord certainly will provide sufficient Grace to bring the patient through the healing process. That we can rest assured that, as Christians who abide in the Lord, we are in safe hands, is evident from another of the author's invaluable books, *Seeing God Through the Human Body*, where we are reminded that "we are fearfully and wonderfully made" (Psalm 139: 14). The intricate design and workings of the human body is a miracle in itself, and of this we are often reminded in this *Christian Health Education Manual*.

The *Manual* is very readable, all the more so on account of the frequent illustrations from the doctor-author's own consulting room. There is the woman, for instance, who comes to him complaining of night sweats and unaccountable swings of mood. In the traditional African context she and others might have thought that the sudden and inexpiable condition pointed to witchcraft. Similarly, the sudden inexplicable death of a successful businessman who appeared to be robust and healthy might have made Africans in a traditional context suspect, again, the wiles of a witch doctor. The author, however, shows how both of these instances are explained by established medical science—the onset of menopause, in the case of the woman, and high blood pressure, which is often undetected, in the case of the businessman.

The *Manual* is consistent in its logical and methodical structure, where each condition or complaint is explained through a systematic pattern of health risks that might trigger the disease or condition (like breast cancer), causes of the condition (like genetics—it might be an established pattern in the family history), symptoms of the condition or disease, methods of diagnosis (like clinical examination), and principles and methods of treatment or cure.

It is a practical book, and an informative one, too, for if the reader has had any lapse or gap in his or her education or schooling in biology and physiology, this book will bring the reader up to speed in a friendly and even entertaining manner, for this doctor knows how to sweeten the pill, which includes the sweet and loving name of Jesus! Indeed, this is a doctor with an attractive bedside manner, who speaks to the reader not as a superior doctor but as a friend and yet as an equal, never pedantic and never aloof.

What makes the book especially unique, of course, is the perspective of the divine dimension that gives the Christian a special relationship with the Great Designer of his or her body. One possible treatment for menopause in women is HRT treatment (Hormone Replacement Therapy). As followers of Christ the Great Physician, no matter what our malaise might be, we also have the privilege of access to DRT (Divine Replacement Therapy)! Indeed, this Manual comes with the author's sincere prayer that all who read it will be blessed through the replacement of unbelief with positive faith in the unlimited power of Jesus of Nazareth.

Charles Muller
Diadem Books
MA (Wales), PhD (London), D.Litt (UFS), D.Ed (SA)

INTRODUCTION

THE ORIGIN OF DISEASE

S omeone may ask: why come out with a health education manual? After all, there are several such manuals on the market—both in the traditional as well as the online bookshops. One can also read about matters relating to health and healthy living on the internet, in health magazines, as well as in the popular press.

I am not disputing this. The fact remains, however, that the majority of material on health matters on the market are written by individuals who either do not believe that you and I were created by Almighty God, or even if they do, fail to take what I will term the "Divine factor" into account when dealing with the issue relating to our health.

This book will adopt a different approach, by tracing the origin of disease to its very root—yes, to its very origin. It is only when we get to the very bottom of this, the reason for or cause of disease, that we can, in my opinion, effectively prevent it; and even if we are not able to do so, adopt the right approach aimed at cure.

Why is mankind afflicted with disease in the first place?

Why, for example, is it that *Vibrio cholerae* bacteria, that minute organism which is visible only under the microscope, is permitted to attack the human being to bring about the disease cholera, which is characterised by symptoms such as diarrhoea, vomiting and resultant dehydration, a condition which, untreated, leads to certain death?

Why is it that the virus associated with the now well-known disease HIV/AIDS is allowed to infect the human being in the first place?

Let me take the matter to another level. Why is it that a human being can become so infuriated as to pick up a gun and shoot another human being, to inflict life-threatening injuries—a condition that necessitates (where the facilities are available) the urgent despatch of an Ambulance that speeds through our streets, siren blaring and blue lights flashing, to pick up and conduct the victim to the A&E department? The hapless victim, or patient, might then be whisked to the operating theatre and operated on by willing and keen staff intent on rescuing him or her form almost certain death.

That single act of the infuriated human being might now engage dozens, if not more, hospital staff in the following days, if not weeks, even months, as they struggle to repair the damage that the single burst of anger has inflicted on a fellow human being. Why was the individual who inflicted this suffering and train of events so infuriated in the first place?

Medical science has identified the viruses, bacteria and parasites that cause the various diseases, but why they are permitted to attack you and me in the first place, is a question it cannot answer. While it may try to treat the symptoms of the problem, the very root cause of the disorder on the other hand is not tackled.

Before I proceed any further, please come with me, dear reader, to the Book of Genesis. You may want to read the whole of Genesis, chapters 1 to 3. For the sake of space, however, I will here reproduce only some passages from that portion of scripture:

In the beginning God created the heaven and the earth.
Genesis 1:1

And God said, Let us make man in our image, after our likeness: and let them have dominion over the fish of the sea, and over the fowl of the air, and over the cattle, and over all the earth, and over every creeping thing that creepeth upon the earth.

So God created man in his own image, in the image of God created he him; male and female created he them.

And God blessed them, and God said unto them, Be fruitful, and multiply, and replenish the earth, and subdue it: and have dominion over the fish of the sea, and over the fowl of the air, and over every living thing that moveth upon the earth. Genesis 1: 26-28

And God saw everything that he had made, and, behold, it was very good. And the evening and the morning were the sixth day. Genesis 1:31

And the LORD God commanded the man, saying, Of every tree of the garden thou mayest freely eat: But of the tree of the knowledge of good and evil, thou shalt not eat of it: for in the day that thou eatest thereof thou shalt surely die. Genesis 2:16-17

Now the serpent was more subtil than any beast of the field which the LORD God had made. And he said unto the woman, Yea, hath God said, Ye shall not eat of every tree of the garden? And the woman said unto the serpent, We may eat of the fruit of the trees of the garden:

But of the fruit of the tree which is in the midst of the garden, God hath said, Ye shall not eat of it, neither shall ye touch it, lest ye die.

And the serpent said unto the woman, Ye shall not surely die: For God doth know that in the day ye eat thereof, then your eyes shall be opened, and ye shall be as gods, knowing good and evil.

And when the woman saw that the tree was good for food, and that it was pleasant to the eyes, and a tree to be desired to make one wise, she took of the fruit thereof, and did eat, and gave also unto her husband with her; and he did eat.

And the eyes of them both were opened, and they knew that they were naked; and they sewed fig leaves together, and made themselves aprons.

And they heard the voice of the LORD God walking in the garden in the cool of the day: and Adam and his wife hid themselves from the presence of the LORD God amongst the trees of the garden.

And the LORD God called unto Adam, and said unto him, Where art thou? And he said, I heard thy voice in the garden, and I was afraid, because I was naked; and I hid myself. And he said, Who told thee that thou wast naked? Hast thou eaten of the tree, whereof I commanded thee that thou shouldest not eat?

And the man said, The woman whom thou gavest to be with me, she gave me of the tree, and I did eat.

And the LORD God said unto the woman, What is this that thou hast done? And the woman said, The serpent beguiled me, and I did eat.

And the LORD God said unto the serpent, Because thou hast done this, thou art cursed above all cattle, and above every beast of the field; upon thy belly shalt thou go, and dust shalt thou eat all the days of thy life:

And I will put enmity between thee and the woman, and between thy seed and her seed; it shall bruise thy head, and thou shalt bruise his heel.

Unto the woman he said, I will greatly multiply thy sorrow and thy conception; in sorrow thou shalt bring forth children; and thy desire shall be to thy husband, and he shall rule over thee.

And unto Adam he said, Because thou hast hearkened unto the voice of thy wife, and hast eaten of the tree, of which I commanded thee, saying, Thou shalt not eat of it: cursed is the ground for thy sake; in sorrow shalt thou eat of it all the days of thy life.

Thorns also and thistles shall it bring forth to thee; and thou shalt eat the herb of the field;

In the sweat of thy face shalt thou eat bread, till thou return unto the ground; for out of it wast thou taken: for dust thou art, and unto dust shalt thou return. Genesis 3:1-19

The above verses of scripture will form the cornerstone of much of the discussions in this book. Indeed, the Fall of Mankind in the Garden of Eden and the subsequent curse pronounced on Mankind by Almighty God in the Garden of Eden will be the foundation on which much of the discussions in this book will be based. For without the Fall of our original parents, Adam and Eve, there would be no diseases, no suffering, no death. There would be no hospitals, no health centres, no pharmacies. The professions of the nurse, the pharmacist, the dentist, the doctor and other health care providers would indeed all be superfluous but for the events recorded in Genesis Chapter 3.

From the above verses of scripture we learn the following:

1) Human Beings were created by Almighty God, in His image.
2) At the very beginning, when Almighty God created the Universe, everything was perfect—there was no disease, no suffering, no death.
3) Disease, suffering and death came into the world as a result of the curse pronounced on Adam and Eve after they had disobeyed Almighty God.
4) Almighty God made a promise of redemption in the verse:

And I will put enmity between thee and the woman, and between thy seed and her seed; it shall bruise thy head, and thou shalt bruise his heel. Genesis 3:15

The promised Redeemer is the Lord Jesus Christ. He was not only to lead us back to the Lord but also to heal our diseases and ailments:

Surely he hath born our griefs, and carried our sorrows: yet we did esteem him stricken, smitten of God, and afflicted.
But he was wounded for our transgressions, he was bruised for our iniquities: the chastisement of our peace was upon him; and with his stripes we are healed. Isaiah 53:4&5

I want to emphasise point number 3:

Disease, suffering and death came into the world as a result of the curse pronounced on Adam and Eve after they had disobeyed Almighty God.

Though Almighty God in His mercy devised a plan of salvation after the fall of Adam and Eve, Divine judgement on Adam and Eve, once pronounced, had to stand as it is.

So shall my word be that goeth forth out of my mouth: it shall not return unto me void, but it shall accomplish that which I please, and it shall prosper in the thing whereto I sent it. Isaiah 55:11

Thus, though we are promised healing through the stripes of the Lord Jesus Christ, disease as such was not to leave us, at least as far as this fallen world exists.

There are some Christians who, probably based on the promise of Isaiah 53:5, completely reject any form of medical treatment on falling sick.

While not trying to be a judge on others, I solemnly beg to differ from these brothers and sisters in Christ. We are indeed to pray for healing from diseases, any kind of disease. That should not, for example, prevent us from injecting insulin in case we suffer from diabetes, a condition that will be dealt with in some detail later in the book. After all, who created insulin but Almighty God? What medical science over the years has discovered is the mechanism by which insulin regulates blood sugar levels in the body—nothing else.

Medical science did not place insulin in our bodies in the first place. It only employs the knowledge gained in the build-up and function of the glucose-regulator for our common good.

If you have prayed to the Lord to heal you of diabetes, I believe one hundred per cent that He can indeed intervene in your situation. We do however know from scripture that sometimes He tarries a while. You may, for reasons that you and I as ordinary human beings cannot fathom, not experience healing at all. That does not, in my opinion, mean that He does not love you.

In Isaiah 55:8 & 9 we read:

For my thoughts are not your thoughts, neither are your ways my ways, saith the LORD.
For as the heavens are higher than the earth, so are my ways higher than your ways, and my thoughts than your thoughts.

In 2 Corinthians 12:7-9 Apostle Paul wrote:

And lest I should be exalted above measure through the abundance of the revelations, there was given to me a thorn in the flesh, the messenger of Satan to buffet me, lest I should be exalted above measure.

For this thing I besought the Lord thrice, that it might depart from me. And he said unto me, My grace is sufficient for thee: for my strength is made perfect in weakness. Most gladly therefore will I rather glory in my infirmities, that the power of Christ may rest upon me.

In the above passage it is generally believed that the Apostle Paul spoke about a disease (many think it was an eye condition) that was not healed by the Lord.

So I urge you to keep on praying to the Lord for the healing of your diabetes. You may from time to time, depending on your faith, perhaps decide to skip your treatment for a day, test your blood sugar levels regularly during the course of the day to establish whether they are normal without treatment.

Should the blood sugar begins to rise without treatment, I would advise that you return to your medication and continue praying. Yes, keep on praying; pray indeed without ceasing, for I know no weapon at the disposal of a Christian but prayer.

Yes, I do believe that prayer and conventional medical science do not contravene each other. Indeed, they can and should co-operate wonderfully in our battle against disease. Indeed, when you and I sit down to consider all that can, for example, go wrong when we go to the hospital to have what the doctors describe as a routine procedure to remove an inflamed appendix, we will recognise the need for prayer at every stage of our stay.

However, someone may well counter my assertion by pointing to the fact that doctors who are atheists perform surgery on patients who are atheists with good results. I am not disputing that fact. What such individuals, yes, such avowed atheists may not realise, even though they are at war with their Maker, is that He may nevertheless extend his favours towards them.

But I say unto you, Love your enemies, bless them that curse you, do good to them that hate you, and pray for them which despitefully use you, and persecute you; That ye may be the children of your Father which is in heaven: for he maketh his sun to rise on the evil and on the good, and sendeth rain on the just and on the unjust. Matthew 5: 44 & 45

Having said that by way of introduction, I shall now to proceed to tackle the task I have set for myself, namely to educate Christians in particular and the public at large about how to prevent and also treat some of the common diseases that afflict us as a result of the factors already touched on.

PROLOGUE

"My People Perish For Lack Of Knowledge"

∞

My people are destroyed for lack of knowledge: because thou hast rejected knowledge, I will also reject thee, that thou shalt be no priest to me: seeing thou hast forgotten the law of thy God, I will also forget thy children. Hosea 4:6

A s already mentioned, the goal of this book is to educate—to provide the reader with a broad knowledge about the causes and treatment of some of the common diseases that afflict Humanity.

I want to stress what I just said—the aim of the book is to educate. It is by no means therefore meant to incite fear or apprehension in the reader. I appeal to you, dear reader, not to be anxious if you think you may be displaying symptoms of a particular disease touched on in the book. Remember the words of our Lord Jesus Christ:

These things I have spoken unto you, that in me ye might have peace. In the world ye shall have tribulation: but be of good cheer; I have overcome the world. John 16:33

Whatever situations that may face us as Christians—diseases, emotional trauma, poverty, job loss—we are to bring them before the Throne of Grace and rest assured the Good Lord will help us sort them out.

Indeed, there is the need for us to educate ourselves concerning several aspects of our life, in particular in regard to matters relating to our health.

My people are destroyed for lack of knowledge: because thou hast rejected knowledge, I will also reject thee, that thou shalt be no priest to me: seeing thou hast forgotten the law of thy God, I will also forget thy children. Hosea 4:6

Based on the experience I have gained as a family doctor, I have come to realise that many, including Christians, lack a background knowledge of some of the most common diseases that afflict us.

As Christians we know we are on our way to the Promised Land. We have not got there yet; indeed, we still find ourselves in an imperfect world. We need as a result to inform ourselves, if even on a general basis, about how Almighty God built our body, how it functions, how to prevent and also cure some of the common diseases that can afflict us on account of living in a fallen world.

'My people perish for lack of knowledge.' Lack of knowledge, indeed, can lead us into trouble in several aspects of life, including the area of our health. An example from my own life will serve to illustrate this.

Shortly after becoming a Christian, I received a vision from the Lord that saw me walking on the streets of a strange settlement that turned out to be Europe. Believing this to be the plan of the Lord for my life, I left my native Ghana to work in Nigeria to earn my plane ticket for Europe.[1] Initially the going was very tough for me in Nigeria; I had to do odd jobs on construction sites to survive.

Eventually, I came to live with a group of young men from Amantia, my mother's hometown, in a makeshift accommodation in Shagamu, a town about 50 kilometres to the north of Lagos. Just as in my case, they had all recently arrived in Nigeria in search of work.

Money was a very scarce commodity in the "colony". Soon word went round the settlement to the effect that one could purchase, directly from the butchers, chunks of fat from the cattle slaughtered on a daily basis for almost free. We got excited about the offer. Almost every day a few of us went on an errand to the butchers to purchase considerable amounts of the

---

[1] An account of how the Lord led me from my native Ghana into medical school in Europe may be read in my book *THE CALL THAT CHANGED MY LIFE*, published by Thank You Jesus Books.

cheap animal fat. With it we prepared soup as part of our main evening meal.

I really did enjoy the several chunks of fat apportioned me. Now, looking back, I realise how foolish I was to consume those pieces of pure animal fat! If I had at that time been informed about the health risks of consuming considerable amounts of fat within a short period of time, I would surely have avoided it.

There is a saying that ignorance is a disease. Not only is it a disease, but our ignorance of the causes and symptoms of diseases can lead us to fear, anxiety, sleepless nights and even false accusations and suspicions. Well, readers who have grown up in developed countries in Western Europe and the US may not really appreciate how ignorance about the causes and symptoms of diseases can indeed lead to false accusations and suspicions.

Well, I grew up in a society in which there is a general tendency to attribute to witchcraft, wizards, evil spirits and what have you blame for all the woes, including diseases, especially those that appear mysterious, that might afflict residents there.

I am not in any way implying that I do not believe in the existence of such evil spirits. In as much as I believe, as a Christian, in the existence of Almighty God, do I also believe in the reality of Satan and the hordes of demonic hosts that serve under the great Deceiver. There are certain instances, however, when a lack of knowledge of diseases might lead some to arrive at wrong conclusions as to why they have become victims of those diseases.

I have in mind the case a pastor friend of mine, a case I was told of the other day. It involved a member of his congregation, a woman in her late forties. She came to his counselling and prayer session and complained about the recent onset of the symptoms which appeared very mysterious to her: the sudden onset of hot flushes which could all of sudden turn into a cold feeling, a feeling as if she was walking in the middle of the arctic winter! Her symptoms, following closely on the heels of her discovery that her husband had been cheating on her with a comparatively younger woman, led her to conclude (not even suspect) that her rival had visited a 'jujuman' to cast a spell on her.

Much as I do not condone the selfish and despicable act of the younger lady trying, as it were, to snatch her husband from her, she would perhaps not have come to that conclusion if she had been informed about menopause and the possible symptoms associated with it! Indeed, if she had not been ignorant about menopause and the possible symptoms that can accompany it, she would have prayed to the Lord to help ease her symptoms instead of becoming alarmed and apportioning others the blame for her malaise.

So, dear Christian friends, we have to educate ourselves. Being a Christian does not mean we have to be ignorant about things that affect our lives. As Tony Blair, a former Prime Minister of the UK once emphasised, "Education, Education, Education!" Yes education matters, especially in matters affecting our health.

PART 1

PREVENTION IS BETTER THAN CURE

Chapter 1

Disease Prevention through Godly Living

∽

Prevention is better than cure—that is a well-known saying. For example, instead of treating a patient with full blown clinical symptoms of cholera, it is better in the first place to provide the individual with clean drinking water, clean sanitation and also to educate the individual about the need to maintain good personal hygiene.

He who is not sick needs no physician. Let us pause a moment and consider our world suddenly transformed into a world free of disease—yes, a world populated only by healthy individuals. Imagine that—a world of healthy people where there is no diabetes, no arthritis, no HIV, no malaria, no mental illness, no cancer! Arguably, the number of the unemployed would suddenly shoot up into the high heavens resulting in possible social unrest as all our hospitals, policlinics, health centres and psychiatric institutions closed their doors and sent their entire staff home for lack of work!

We Christians believe that in the world to come, there will indeed be no disease, no suffering and—no death! But so long as we are resident in a fallen and evil world, we will continue to be plagued with diseases. So I do urge all those aspiring to become nurses, pharmacists, dentists, doctors, psychiatrists, not to lose heart, for indeed as long as the world exists in its present state there will be plenty of work for you!

Still, there is the need for each and every one of us as individuals to do whatever we can to prevent disease. This brings to mind what I learnt from my driving school teacher in the northern German city of Hanover several years ago. He taught his driving class that three factors come into play the moment a driver joins the flow of traffic. These are:

1) The driving skills of the individual involved.
2) The condition of the vehicle he or she is driving.
3) The other drivers on the road, the condition of the road and the elements.

Whereas one can influence the first two factors, our teacher pointed out, the individual is completely at a loss as to third factor. He urged us always to do all we could do to minimise the chances of becoming involved in a road traffic accident by positively influencing the first two factors. For example, we should never drive under the influence of alcohol or when we are too tired, or too unwell to do so.

Concerning the second factor, he advised us always to make sure the vehicle we are driving is in perfect condition—with properly functioning brakes, good tyres, well-functioning lighting systems, etc.

In a sense, that thinking can also apply to the area of our health. It is said that the best defence is attack. In the area of medicine, I will modify that saying to this: the best cure is prevention! So let us make this our highest priority—the prevention of disease.

What kind of prevention, one might ask? Well, many a reader is surely aware of some of the well-known disease-preventive measures around. We read of them in books on health education; they may be handed to us when we visit our family doctor; we may also read about them from health education journals and the popular press.

These include maintaining good personal hygiene, drinking clean water, having vaccinations, and taking prophylaxis such as malaria tablets prior to travelling to the tropics, etc. Later in the discussion I will also touch on disease-preventive measures such as eating a balanced diet and exercising the body on a regular basis.

Many a Christian will agree that our Lord Jesus Christ is the great physician of all times. We do indeed read in the Bible that He healed the blind, the deaf, the dumb, the paralysed. In other words, He actively intervened to heal diseases.

But have we sat down to consider the area of prevention? Have we ever linked Dr Jesus, the Great Physician of all time, with preventive medicine? Indeed, have we, as followers of the Great High Priest, sat down to consider the huge disease-preventing potential of the Word of God?

It might indeed not have occurred to you, but it is indeed true that the mere adherence to the teachings of our Lord and Saviour Jesus Christ, either spoken directly by Himself, or through inspiration by His servants, could avert several diseases.

I want to stress my point. We may indeed not be able to prevent every kind of disease afflicting fallen Mankind, by accepting and abiding by the Word of Scripture. Still, it is my deep conviction that we could indeed avert many kinds of diseases, not only those affecting the body, but also those affecting the mind if we would accept and keep to the teachings of the Good Shepherd.

Modern medical science will not tell you that, because, after all, it is scientific-based and atheistically oriented. This book, as the title suggests, is meant in the first place for Christians, so I will take the privilege upon myself to point out the facts as I see them. You may not agree with me on everything I say, of course. Well, I do not claim to be the last authority in anything. I am merely trying to express my thinking with a good conscience, based on my knowledge and experience as a Christian doctor.

Now let us consider this passage of scripture attributed to the Lord Himself:

Therefore I say unto you, Take no thought for your life, what ye shall eat, or what ye shall drink; nor yet for your body, what ye shall put on. Is not the life more than meat, and the body than raiment?

Behold the fowls of the air: for they sow not, neither do they reap, nor gather into barns; yet your heavenly Father feedeth them. Are ye not much better than they? Which of you by taking thought can add one cubit unto his stature?

And why take ye thought for raiment? Consider the lilies of the field, how they grow; they toil not, neither do they spin: And yet I say unto you, That even Solomon in all his glory was not arrayed like one of these.

Wherefore, if God so clothe the grass of the field, which today is, and tomorrow is cast into the oven, shall he not much more clothe you, O ye of little faith?

Therefore take no thought, saying, What shall we eat? or, What shall we drink? or, Wherewithal shall we be clothed? (For after all these things do the Gentiles seek:) for your heavenly Father knoweth that ye have need of all these things.

But seek ye first the kingdom of God, and his righteousness; and all these things shall be added unto you. Take therefore no thought for the morrow: for the morrow shall take thought for the things of itself. Sufficient unto the day is the evil thereof. Matthew 6:25-34

Note the last verse (6:34) especially: **'Take therefore no thought for the morrow: for the morrow shall take thought for the things of itself. Sufficient unto the day is the evil thereof.'**

A close look at the sentence as it stands, indeed, a close reflection on the verse as it stands, will probably lead one to ask the question: 'Why did we have to wait for the Lord to tell us something that, in reality, is a matter of common sense?'

The definition of *tomorrow* is—'the day following (or after) today.' Now, as we are living today, the day following today has not yet arrived, has it? We are indeed always living in the *today*! Why then do you and I allow the problems of tomorrow, yes, the day after today, to burden us, to cause us a headache today? Today is *today*; tomorrow never comes—it's as simple as that!

And yet how often do we permit the problems of tomorrow to weigh on our brains, yes, to burden us to the extent that some of us eventually end up on the psychiatric ward!

Let us take a concrete example—the threat of job loss. That could lead to anxious thoughts—how we will feed ourselves and our family, how we will pay our utility bills, how we will pay our rent or mortgage, and how that might lead to the repossession of our homes, etc.

As the fear of the possible loss of our job tomorrow (tomorrow, that in effect never comes) persists, so also would the thickness of the dark cloud of despair surrounding us increase, to the extent it could lead us to consider ending it all!

We may indeed still have our jobs—only the *threat* of losing it might be looming over our heads. Still, we suffer anxiety and sleep disturbance as a result.

Now the Lord Jesus Christ is not saying that we should not make the effort to avert the situation. We may for example apply for other jobs. We could also consider the possibility of becoming self- employed. What He is urging us is to do our best in the situation and leave the rest to Him. Our efforts, backed by our prayers, can change the situation, whereas our anxiety, sleep disturbance and depression cannot.

I am not implying that I am immune to that human weakness. I have indeed harboured anxious thoughts in the past. It did not lead to full blown depression but they were nevertheless anxious thoughts that occupied me for a while. Now, looking back on those periods in my life, how silly indeed was I to have harboured those thoughts!

Indeed, if only we could accept those words of the Lord with childlike faith, how many problems that plague us—anxiety, tension headaches, sleep disturbance, depression, would be averted.

Let me move on to another passage of scripture:

> *Know ye not that your bodies are the members of Christ? shall I then take the members of Christ, and make them the members of an harlot? God forbid. What? know ye not that he which is joined to an harlot is one body? for two, saith he, shall be one flesh. But he that is joined unto the Lord is one spirit.*
>
> *Flee fornication. Every sin that a man doeth is without the body; but he that committeth fornication sinneth against his own body.*
>
> *What? know ye not that your body is the temple of the Holy Ghost which is in you, which ye have of God, and ye are not your own?*
>
> *For ye are bought with a price: therefore glorify God in your body, and in your spirit, which are God's. 1 Corinthians 6: 15-20*

I want us to consider in particular Versus 19 & 20:

> *What? know ye not that your body is the temple of the Holy Ghost which is in you, which ye have of God, and ye are not your own?*
> *For ye are bought with a price: therefore glorify God in your body, and in your spirit, which are God's.*

Now the Holy Spirit through the Apostle Paul is telling us that our respective bodies represent the TEMPLE of the Holy Spirit! I want us to pause for a moment to ponder over this statement. I really do have the impression that often we take our responsibility as Christians too lightly. Wherein lies the problem, friends? Is it because the message coming out of the pulpit these days is made up of things like: "Pay your tithes and receive your blessings", "May the Lord bless you and prosper you", "All things work together for good"—without also including "We are Soldiers of the Cross", "God is a spirit and those who worship him should worship him in spirit and in truth", "Your bodies are a temple of the Holy Spirit," etc?

"Your body is a temple of the Holy Spirit"—that is an awesome statement. I am not trying to be scary, but, indeed, sometimes I am even afraid to call myself a Christian because it is indeed a very high calling—indeed, it is.

Now the Holy Father has sent His Holy spirit to dwell in us. As real soldiers of the Cross, our bodies are no longer ours, but the Lord's. This is an amazing fact. Now we know that the Lord is Holy and nothing impure can come near Him. So if the Holy Spirit is dwelling in us, then nothing impure should come near our body to render it impure. It's as if we are wearing a snow white wedding gown—so dirt, filth, impurity, away, away with you! Go away, all impurity—never come near me!

When I was young, when I at certain times became angry with my parents, I decided to go without food. Why did I do that? Well, in my immature mind I thought I was punishing them!

In the same vein we might think *we* may be doing the Lord a favour, i.e. manipulating Him, by heeding (or not heeding!) his admonition to us to keep our, yes, the temple of the Holy Spirit, pure. If that is what we think, then please let us discard those ideas at this very moment as we read these lines!

This leads me to consider some of the diseases we could catch if we choose to introduce dirt or impurity into the temple of the Living God that we are.

SMOKING

If my body is the temple of the Holy Spirit then I will not pollute it by smoking. Please do not get me wrong. I am not implying that if you smoke, you are not a child of God. It is possible that you acquired your habit before becoming a Christian. As the saying goes, habits, once acquired, are difficult to break. My prayer to the Lord for you is that you will be able to overcome your habit.

For those who have not acquired that habit, however, my advice is: hands off the potential pollutant of the temple of the Living God!

You will not save only money by not smoking, you will also avert the risk of contracting any of the diseases associated with smoking—lung cancer, heart and circulatory problems, lung emphysema, etc.

What some men are not aware of is this—by affecting the blood vessels of the body, including the small vessels (capillaries), smoking can also have a detrimental effect on your ability to perform as a man. Why allow smoking to impair your ability to perform one aspect of your conjugal rights as husband as instituted by Almighty God?

ALCOHOL

Woe unto them that rise up early in the morning, that they may follow strong drink; that continue until night, till wine inflame them! Isaiah 5:11

One day as I worked as a prison doctor in the UK, a highly respected medical doctor came to prison on remand. His offence? Here we go:

1) Under the influence of alcohol he threatened to kill his wife and their two daughters with a kitchen knife.
2) Scared to death, the threatened wife called the police. Moments later the sirens of the approaching police vehicles filled the air. Before their arrival, the drunken man ran into the street, armed with the kitchen knife.
3) Soon he came across a young woman about to board her vehicle. With his knife pointing at the frightened lady, he demanded that she hand him the car keys. Soon he was fleeing away from the police in the "stolen" vehicle. The police gave chase.
4) As he fled he rammed the vehicle into several other parked cars on the street. In the end he was arrested.
5) At the time I met him, he was on a 24-hour watch due to the threat of suicide.

The solicitors and experts of the law among us may want to sit down to list the number of possible offences committed by this learned and noble fellow. Indeed, when I met him, I just could not imagine that the decent looking individual sitting before me could commit the offences he was charged with. He himself, now freed from the influence of alcohol, could also not fathom what he had done.

Alcohol—what havoc it can cause! As in the case of smoking, I am not implying that consuming alcohol does not make you a child of God.

As far as I am concerned, alcohol has never been a problem. Indeed, even before I decided to follow the Lord, I hardly drank alcohol. Since becoming a Christian I have on very, very rare instances drank sips of alcohol, for instance, to share in the toast of a departing colleague at work. As I write, I do not remember the last time I tasted alcohol—ten years ago, perhaps? At the moment, I just do not see the need to do so.

Well, you may read in the newspaper or elsewhere that alcohol, when consumed in moderation, may help prevent certain types of heart diseases. I am not disputing a conclusion arrived at by way of careful clinical study.

The emphasis is on *moderate* usage, for the same alcohol, if consumed in considerable amounts over a long period of time, can also lead to what the doctors term alcoholic cardiomyopathy, a diseases of the heart muscles that can lead to heart failure and death.

As the above examples illustrate, it is not the Lord who will benefit from our decision either not to drink alcohol at all or to do so only occasionally and in moderation.

If we do not heed the warning in Isaiah 5:11 and decide to pollute the temple of the Holy Spirit with alcohol, we may well end of up like that noble and respectable doctor. Even if we don't sink to his level of degradation and loss of control, however, we could nevertheless cause harm to our body through the excessive and long-term consumption of alcohol. I have already described the adverse effect it could cause to the heart muscles.

The organ most likely to be damaged by alcohol is the liver. Perhaps you are not fully aware of why the Creator placed the liver in our body. Well, as I mentioned in my book *SEEING GOD THROUGH THE HUMAN BODY*, the liver is one of the most sophisticated factories around. Its main function is to detoxify, or make harmless, harmful substances, including alcohol, that get into our body. Now if we, through alcohol, cause harm to the organ responsible for detoxifying harmful substances that get into our body, the implication must be clear to us.

Another important organ of the body that can adversely be affected by alcohol is the pancreas. When we come to look at diabetes in some detail, we will learn that it is the pancreas that produce insulin. Now alcohol could damage the pancreas and lead, among other things, to diabetes.

Apart from the above, alcohol can also adversely affect our brain, nerves, gullet and stomach. Alcohol consumption can also have a negative impact on the outcome of a pregnancy.

ILLICIT DRUG USE

In some countries, especially the western industrialised nations, the impact on the health of the body as well as the socio-economic impact of the use of drugs such as cannabis, cocaine, heroin, amphetamine, etc., is enormous. I do not want delve into details about the problem of illicit drug use, a topic that will require volumes to treat.

It is indeed my fervent prayer that you, my dear reader, your family members, friends, acquaintance or anyone dear to your heart, will never, never become entrapped, either directly or indirectly, by the monsters that enslave so many—heroin, cocaine, cannabis, or whatever drug of addiction there is on the market. That indeed is my heartfelt prayer.

SEXUAL IMPURITY

Just before the Apostle Paul mentioned that our body is the temple of the Holy Spirit, he touched on something that makes me wonder whether he had some medical training himself. If that is not the case, as it is generally believed, then for sure the Holy Spirit gave him real insight into medical conditions.

Now the Apostle states in 1 Corithians 6: 18:

'Flee fornication. Every sin that a man doeth is without the body; but he that committeth fornication sinneth against his own body.'

Just as in the case of the substances I dealt with earlier, the Apostle Paul is telling us that we do Almighty God no favour by keeping to His rules in regard to sexual purity. On the contrary, it is our own body we preserve from exposure to all kinds of diseases. That leads me to the area of sexually transmitted diseases, or STDs for short.

Before I proceed, allow me to make an observation. Sex is a gift from God. No human being invented it. None of our scientists—Einstein, Newton, Faraday, just the beginning of a long list of names, indeed, the best brains that we can think of—whether they believe in God or not; whether they are Nobel prize winners or not; yes indeed, the most brilliant among the brilliants of our race, past, present or in the future, is capable of inventing the concept of sexual reproduction, in this case human sexual reproduction.

Only the King of Kings and Lord of Lords, the Great High Priest, the 'I am' that 'I Am', the one and only High God, could do it. Join me, ladies and gentlemen, in bowing our heads to our Lord who indeed deserves our praise. Human Sexuality is a gift of God to Humankind. It was given on a certain condition, however:

Therefore shall a man leave his father and his mother, and shall cleave unto his wife: and they shall be one flesh. And they were both naked, the man and his wife, and were not ashamed. Genesis 2:24-25

As you and I know, this beautiful gift of Almighty God to Mankind has in the meantime been corrupted to the high heavens.

Dear reader, you might have, like the author of these lines, been living according to the dictates of the flesh. Now that we are born again, please let us let the past be the past and let us strive for holiness in the Lord.

Yes indeed, if by God's grace, we have come to see the light, let us dwell in the light; yes, let us crucify the flesh and all the lust associated with it.

To the very young ones, those who have been fortunate to see that Light at a young age, I plead with you to strive for high ideals, also in the area of your sexual life. The ideal you should strive for is to avoid sex unless in marriage. It is an ideal worth pursuing, so strive to attain it. You may in the end miss your set goal; nevertheless it is worth striving for. No, do not give up at the very beginning with words like, "It is not easy; it is not practicable." Some have managed to make it, so pursue it with all vigour. I pray the Lord to provide the needed willpower to help you endure.

Apostle Paul writes in Philippians 4:13,

"I can do all things through Christ who strengthens me."

We are indeed overcomers in the mighty name of the our Lord and Saviour Jesus Christ.

The Christian life is indeed worthy of displaying the highest discipline and strongest degree of willpower in our sexual life. Apart from saving ourselves the risk of contracting some of the diseases I am about to touch on, we will also preserve ourselves from problems such as a broken heart, disappointment, depression, unwanted pregnancy, etc.

The sexual pleasure we enjoy for a few minutes could indeed lead to days, weeks, months, even years of regret, remorse, guilt, acrimony, etc.

The other day I met a man in prison who told me he was cheating on his wife. At one stage he had problems which bothered him, relating to money his girlfriend demanded. In the end she entrapped him and accused him of rape. Eventually he received a long sentence. His cheating on his wife having been exposed, she divorced him. Lingering in prison, he regretted his actions to the high heavens. He yearned for his wife and longed to have his children back—too late, it seemed.

> *But if ye will not do so, behold, ye have sinned against the LORD: and be sure your sin will find you out.Numbers 32:23*

It is worthy of note that often it is not the Lord who finds us out, but rather it is our sins.

The Lord indeed may forgive us when we pray about our failings, but will the bacteria, the virus, the fungi, etc?

It is indeed in our interest to swim against the tide of society rather than with it.

> *Enter ye in at the strait gate: for wide is the gate, and broad is the way, that leadeth to destruction, and many there be which go in thereat: Because strait is the gate, and narrow is the way, which leadeth unto life, and few there be that find it. Matthew 7: 13&14*
>
> *Flee fornication. Every sin that a man doeth is without the body; but he that committeth fornication sinneth against his own body. 1 Corinthians 6:18*

The Apostle Paul is probably implying that if we commit sexual sin, we could pray to the Lord for forgiveness. The Lord may forgive us, for He forgives the contrite heart; not so the world of the micro-organism. That in the end could lead to one or more of the following diseases: Chlamydian, Gonorrhoea, HIV, Herpes genitalis, Genital Warts, Syphilis.

I will treat each of the above conditions later on in the book.

BITTERNESS, MALICE, AN UNFORGIVING SPIRIT

For if ye forgive men their trespasses, your heavenly Father will also forgive you: But if ye forgive not men their trespasses, neither will your Father forgive your trespasses. Matthew 6:14-15

Then came Peter to him, and said, Lord, how oft shall my brother sin against me, and I forgive him? till seven times?

Jesus saith unto him, I say not unto thee, Until seven times: but, until seventy times seven. Matthew 18: 21-22

Take heed to yourselves: If thy brother trespass against thee, rebuke him; and if he repent, forgive him. And if he trespass against thee seven times in a day, and seven times in a day turn again to thee, saying, I repent; thou shalt forgive him. Luke 17:3-4

Be ye angry, and sin not: let not the sun go down upon your wrath: Neither give place to the devil. Ephesians 4:26-27

Let all bitterness, and wrath, and anger, and clamour, and evil speaking, be put away from you, with all malice: And be ye kind one to another, tender-hearted, forgiving one another, even as God for Christ's sake hath forgiven you. Ephesians 4:31-32

The New Testament is full of passages that call for forgiveness. In fact, the Gospel of Christ might well be summed up as a Gospel of Forgiveness, Hope, Love and Salvation.

When it comes to the issue of forgiveness, I must admit that it is not always easy to forgive except for the help of the Holy Spirit.

One day one of my patients told me the story of how one of her best friends had literally snatched her husband from her! You may, dear reader, also be aware of similar incidents. How do you and I preach the message of forgiveness to such an injured soul?

I do admit that in the short-term it may be difficult for you and I to forgive someone who has done evil against us. Still, the goal, at least in the medium and long-term, should be forgiveness.

Perhaps it may require a period of fasting and prayer on our part to attain a state of mind that will put us in a position to do so. We are not required to restore the relationship to the extent that we invite the person involved to our home for a cup of tea or coffee. What I believe is required of us is to attain a state of mind where we do not harbour any bitterness or malice against the individual concerned, a state of mind that places us in a position to wish the person involved well in life if need be.

Indeed, no matter how deeply others might offend us, we are called upon by the Lord of Heaven and earth to forgive.

Of course, the Lord of Creation knew what he was talking about. He placed the immune system in our body to defend the body against the invasion of germs and other parasites. Not only does our immune system defend us against outside invaders; later, when we come to deal with cancer, we will learn that cancer results from normal cells that have turned abnormal and are dividing uncontrollably. The immune system is able to identify these abnormal cells and destroy them, in so doing preventing them from growing into a tumour. Thus a strong immune system does not only prevent infection, but also protects us from developing cancer.

Now it has been established by medical science that bitterness, an unforgiving spirit, hatred, cares, worry, stress, etc., can weaken our immune system—yes, the body defences. You can imagine the situation when the soldiers guarding a city go on strike and decide to retire to bed instead of confronting an invading army!

It should indeed not come as a surprise to us that bitterness, hatred, worry and an unforgiving spirit should have an adverse effect on our immune system. Do you remember the last time you felt offended by someone—your partner, brother, sister, friend, colleague? You felt so angered by the person involved that you spent the whole night grumbling over the incident. Mind you, at the time you were struggling to sleep as a result of your grumblings, the individual concerned might have been fast, fast asleep, and like myself probably snoring very deeply.

That individual might very likely wake up the next day, refreshed by the thorough sleep. You, on the other hand, may well have risen the next day with a dejected face, suffering from the effect of the poor sleep of the previous night.

If only matters would end there! The lack of sleep might eventually lead you to fall asleep behind the wheel of your vehicle as you drive to work or the grocery store, which in turn could lead to an accident, perhaps a severe one. Your life could be spared, but the damage could be enormous. It could even lead to your hospitalisation. You now realise what bitterness and an unforgiving spirit can lead to.

DISEASES BROUGHT ABOUT BY FAMILY BREAKDOWN

But I say unto you, that whosoever shall put away his wife, saving for the cause of fornication, causeth her to commit adultery: and whosoever shall marry her that is divorced committeth adultery. Matthew 5:32

Some may not recognise a direct link between a stable and a harmonious home and good health. It is beyond the realm of this book to delve into detail into a topic that could well fill the pages of a complete book. Those blessed to have grown up in a stable, harmonious home as well as those who, unfortunately, have experienced the very opposite constellation, would bear me out as to the positive and negative effects a stable and a broken home can respectively have on the health and well-being of all involved.

I have over the last several years worked as a prison doctor. In the process I have learnt at first hand a fact that previously was not so clear to me, namely that quite a considerable proportion of those addicted to various forms of drugs came from a broken home.

Admittedly, the issue of drug addiction is a complex one. Several factors indeed usually come into play to explain an individual's path to drug addiction.

Still, the point I am driving home is true, that quite a considerable number of addicts owe their condition to broken marriages. With the family torn apart, the children, as it were, also get torn apart, join the wrong company and eventually end up as addicts.

How then do we prevent that situation? Well, as I mentioned at the outset, this book is written for Christians. I dare, therefore, take the privilege to touch on issues that may not be comfortable to everyone.

All scripture is given by inspiration of God, and is profitable for doctrine, for reproof, for correction, for instruction in righteousness: That the man of God may be perfect, thoroughly furnished unto all good works. 2 Timothy 3:16-17

The Lord Jesus Christ, who we serve, stated categorically in *Matthew 5:32*

But I say unto you, That whosoever shall put away his wife, saving for the cause of fornication, causeth her to commit adultery: and whosoever shall marry her that is divorced committeth adultery.

Now let the Church sit down and ask: how many divorces are granted these days solely on the grounds of one of the spouses becoming unfaithful?
Please, I want to repeat that I am not a judge. If that is the impression created in your mind, then I do not think that is fair. Indeed, I am not doing anything apart from calling for a critical self-examination by the church.
If the Church has not been able to keep to the mark expected of it, it is a sign of its weakness. Instead of attempting to rationalise, yes, find excuses for our failing, it is high time, in my opinion, for the Church of the Living Jesus to go on its knees to beg forgiveness.

If my people, which are called by my name, shall humble themselves, and pray, and seek my face, and turn from their wicked ways; then will I hear from heaven, and will forgive their sin, and will heal their land. 2 Chronicles 7:14

Indeed, it is imperative for the body of Christ to make huge efforts to save the family. Instead of swimming with the tide of society, we are called upon to swim against the tide of time. The Church indeed must guide and guard itself against incorporating norms set by a godless society, a society that has lost its orientation, a society that is not rooted on the solid foundations of the teachings of Christ. The end result of such a failing, of compromising instead of staying firm on solid Christian principles, will for a certainty be the cause of misery.

A breakdown of marriage does not affect only the children. Whatever show the individuals may want to put up for the outside world, deep inside them they are traumatised. This leads back to the issue of the effect of bitterness and an unforgiving spirit on our defence system. The body of Christ, let us make a valiant effort to save our marriages, our homes and in so doing help prevent disease.

MENTAL HEALTH PROBLEMS RESULTING FROM BURDENS

Come unto me, all ye that labour and are heavy laden, and I will give you rest. Take my yoke upon you, and learn of me; for I am meek and lowly in heart: and ye shall find rest unto your souls. For my yoke is easy, and my burden is light. Matthew 11:28-30

We all, in some way, are laden with care, or carry various burdens. Some of us were abused as children; yes, we could have been sexually abused as children. Even though we have become Christians, we may still experience flashbacks. These could eventually lead to depression. Often such flashbacks come at times when we are facing problems, when we are not walking close enough to the Lord. We would be helped if we would draw closer to the Lord, through fellowship, fasting, prayer and Bible reading.

Draw nigh to God, and He will draw nigh to you. James 4:8

DISEASES BROUGHT ABOUT BY CONFLICT, POVERTY, AND UNDERDEVELOPMENT

One might not at first glimpse identify a link between holding to the principles taught by scripture and the prevention of diseases—diseases associated with poverty, under-development and conflict.

Now take a look at these verses of scripture:

> *Then Job arose, and rent his mantle, and shaved his head, and fell down upon the ground, and worshipped, And said, Naked came I out of my mother's womb, and naked shall I return thither: the LORD gave, and the LORD hath taken away; blessed be the name of the LORD. Job 1:20-21*
>
> *For we brought nothing into this world, and it is certain we can carry nothing out. And having food and raiment let us be therewith content. But they that will be rich fall into temptation and a snare, and into many foolish and hurtful lusts, which drown men in destruction and perdition.*
>
> *For the love of money is the root of all evil: which while some coveted after, they have erred from the faith, and pierced themselves through with many sorrows. 1 Timothy 6: 7-10*

We have not got into heaven yet. So long as we live in a fallen world there will be poverty, unrest, conflict, wars, etc. These in turn could lead to malnutrition, starvation, poor sanitation, mass displacement, etc. which in turn could lead to disease, etc.

Perhaps this sounds too simplistic. Still, it is my conviction that if those who have the say in the affairs of this world, if our political leaders, our bankers, stockbrokers, etc., would allow Biblical principles to guide and guard their decisions, actions, transactions, etc., we would help alleviate poverty and underdevelopment and with it help prevent disease.

Charity, they say, begins at home, so I will begin with Africa, my original home. Indeed, if many an African leader would come to realise that "Naked came I out of my mother's womb, and naked shall I return thither," and also that "we brought nothing into this world, and it is certain we can carry nothing out," it might lead them to spend the resources at their disposal towards raising the standards of living of their citizens—provide clean drinking water, improve sanitation, invest in agriculture to provide a balanced diet for their residents, etc.—instead of using resources, in many instances already scarce, to enrich themselves and their cronies.

I am not implying this would completely eradicate or prevent all diseases in their various countries—but even if their good governments contributed to the prevention or alleviation of even 1% of the diseases that plague their citizens, their efforts would be worthwhile.

The argument could be carried further to the international scene—to the front doors of the mighty men and women in Berlin, London, Paris, New York, Washington and elsewhere. Indeed, if they would but allow compassion, the love for the citizens living in their respective countries to reflect on the love they have for residents far away from their borders, we may well avert many conflicts, diseases and suffering.

Before I leave this area which admittedly borders more on big politics than matters relating to health, I want us to take a final look at the following verse of scripture:

Pride goeth before destruction, and an haughty spirit before a fall.
Proverbs 16:18

How many wars have been fought in the past, and will surely be fought in the future because of the pride of leaders and their nations?

I am no prophet of doom, but based on this Bible verse, I really do fear that we are pre-empting our doom. Oh, how proud have we become! We have become so proud in regard to what we have been able to achieve. We boast of our biological, scientific, technical, etc. know-how, to the extent that we trample with sheer impunity on the laws and provisions of Almighty God.

Pride comes before a fall—we have been warned. Let us beware lest our pride lead not only to our downfall as individuals, but also to the downfall of the wider world.

I better move on lest I deviate completely from the topic in hand!

Chapter 2

God Helps those who help themselves

⌇

In the previous chapter, I outlined some of the diseases we could prevent just by living godly lives. Apart from living a godly life, there are measures that we ourselves could adopt to keep healthy. One such measure is diet—that is, paying attention to the type of food we introduce to our body system.

The body needs food for energy and growth. There is the need, however, to eat the right quantity and quality of food. That leads me to the concept of a balanced diet. What is a balanced diet? Before I answer this question, I shall use an illustration based on my own life.

When I was growing up in my little village in Ghana, we usually had a meal made from boiled plantains or yams or cocoyams and kontomire (leaves from the cocoyam plant) sauce for breakfast; and the same type of meal for lunch.

The main meal for the day was the evening meal, *fufu*. *Fufu* is made by pounding boiled cassava, plantain, yam or cocoyam into balls and swallowing small portions of the ball with soup. Meat or fish or both are added to the soup, though for our family meat and fish was a scarce commodity. The larger part of the little meat and fish we could afford was reserved for the adults, especially father.

We did not eat fruit on a daily basis. We had some oranges, peas and bananas, and pineapples growing on our farms—but we enjoyed them only during their seasons.

On the whole, the quantity of food I was privileged to enjoy every day was adequate. Indeed, none of us at home needed to starve. Still, *much as I tried* to grow tall, I did not grow taller than 165cm.

Now my son David is 14 years old as I write. At that age he has already passed the 170cm mark and is growing taller and taller. It is generally believed that the height an individual attains is dependent on the individual's parents as well as environmental factors.

Now as far as the parent factor is concerned, though I am not a tall man, I am nevertheless taller than Rita, my wife. So we can rule out the genetic factor as the cause of David's increasing height.

This brings me back to the issue of a balanced diet. The Lord indeed placed food at our disposal. The various types of foodstuffs at our disposal need however to be eaten in the right proportion to have an optimal effect on our bodies.

As a child, I was fed mostly on carbohydrates. That provided me sufficient energy to allow me to go about my daily activities, including walking a total of four miles to and from school. Without sufficient supply of proteins, vitamins, mineral elements, etc., my body however could not grow optimally.

My son David on his part has been privileged to enjoy not only an abundant supply of the various kinds of foodstuffs needed by the body, but also in proportion favourable to optimal growth.

If you are reading these lines and happen to be living under conditions that make it difficult for you to attain a balanced diet on a daily basis, it is my prayer that the Lord will help improve your lot. For those who can afford it, however, it is important that we strive to achieve a balanced diet every day.

Having said this by way of introduction, I wish to explain the concept of a balanced diet as defined by the experts in that area of human endeavour.

As I mentioned above, our body needs various kinds of food items to grow. These are classified into the following groups: carbohydrates, fat, proteins, vitamins, mineral salts and fibres.

Carbohydrates provide the body with energy. Examples of food rich in carbohydrates are: rice, maize, wheat, yams, plantain, cocoyams, etc.

Proteins on their part are required for growth and repair. They are obtained from fish, meat, beans, etc.

Fat, like carbohydrates, is a source of energy. Some vitamins, known as fat-soluble vitamins, are able to dissolve only in fat.

Vitamins are required in small quantities. They are however invaluable to the body since they help bring about several important reactions that take place in our body. Vitamins can be obtained, among others, from fruit such as oranges, apple, banana, strawberries, etc.

Minerals: Several types of minerals are needed by the body for optimal growth and function. Examples of minerals needed by the body are: iron, calcium, sodium and iodine.

Fibre: Also called roughage or bulk, fibre is necessary to promote the wave-like contractions that move food through the intestine. High fibre foods expand the inside walls of the colon, easing the passage of waste. As fibre passes through the intestine undigested, it absorbs large amounts of water, resulting in a softer and bulkier stool. By helping to form a softer, larger stool, fibre thus helps prevent constipation. Examples of foodstuffs rich in fibre are whole fresh fruits, green leafy vegetables, root vegetables, whole grains beans, etc.

A balanced diet is a diet which contains the above ingredients in the right proportions. As a general rule, such a diet should contain about sixty per cent carbohydrates, twenty per cent protein and twenty per cent fat. Vitamins and minerals, though vital to the functioning of our body, on their part, are required in very small proportions.

Not only are we to eat a healthy and balanced diet, we must also resist the temptation to overfeed ourselves. The saying has it that "too much of anything is bad". When it comes to the food that we supply to our body, one might indeed agree with the above saying.

The body needs a certain amount of energy each day in order to function properly. This energy is expressed in calories. The number of calories in a food depends on the type of food involved. One gram of each of the three main types of food: carbohydrates, fat and proteins provides 4, 9 and 4 calories of energy respectively.

The daily calorie requirement of an individual depends on age, height, weight, gender, and activity level. For example, a soldier who has to undergo strenuous exercises on an almost daily basis will require much more calories per day than someone like myself who spends much of his day working on the computer.

As a starting point a female adult with low activity levels requires on the average 2000 calories to maintain a desirable weight, whereas her male adult counterpart with a similar activity level requires about 2,700 calories per day for the same purpose.

People who consume more calories than they burn off in normal daily activity are more likely to be overweight. The reason is that the body converts the extra energy into fat for further storage.

We can indeed draw a parallel with money. In daily life, the majority of us struggle to make ends meet financially. Some, however, manage to obtain those pieces of paper and coins that have been produced by countries to serve as a medium of exchange in surplus—indeed, in some cases in real abundance. Instead of carrying the surplus bank notes and coins around in bags, cartons, suitcases, etc., they choose to deposit them in banks. Usually the banks are able to keep them safe, until perhaps the next credit crunch sets in to threaten them.

There is an important difference between the excess food we eat and the excess money we possess! Whereas we can deposit the excess money in the bank or donate it to charity, for purposes far away from our homes, we can neither deposit the extra fat built up in us outside our body nor donate some to an individual dying of starvation somewhere on our common planet. So in due course we become overweight! We can, as it were, afford to become a little overweight. Beyond a certain limit, however, the additional weight can lead to a horde of health problems. Among other things, it can increase our risk of developing diabetes, high blood pressure, cardiovascular (heart and circulatory) diseases, etc.

On the issue of an ideal weight, one may well ask the question: what then is an ideal weight? There is not a general consensus among the experts in the matter as to what exactly is the ideal weight of an individual. In this book, I will reproduce two of the common references in use.

Broca Index:

This index originated from Paul Broca, a French surgeon, in 1871. It calculates an ideal weight in terms of the height and weight of the individual. The Broca Index defines an ideal weight as follows:

Ideal Weight (in kg) = Height (in cm) – 100, plus or minus 15% for women or 10% for men.

Following this formula, the ideal weight for Miss Eve, 160cm in height, would be between 52kg and 69kg. Mr Adam, boasting the same height as Miss Eve, on his part, would have an ideal weight between 54kg and 66kg.

BMI Index:

Others resort to the more complicated **BMI** or Body Mass index whereby a BMI is calculated based on the formula:

BMI = mass (kg) / height^2 (m^2) for the metric-system, or
BMI = mass (lb) $\times$ 703 / height^2 (inches^2) for the imperial.

Still using Miss Eve as an example: Assuming at a height of 160cm she is found to weigh 80kg, her BMI would be $80/(1.6 \times 1.6) = 31.25$ and would be classified as obese.

BMI	Interpretation
BMI 18.5 to 25	Normal or optimal weight
BMI > 25	Overweight
BMI < 18.5	Underweight
BMI < 17.5	Extremely underweight
BMI = 30 or BMI > 30	Obese
BMI = 40 or BMI > 40	Morbid obesity

You may perhaps wish to use the above formula to calculate your BMI and then determine whether you are, perhaps, heading towards the category 'morbid obese'.

I hasten to add that the above information is provided to educate, not to scare! I believe that with a certain degree of self-discipline, most of us would be in a position to maintain a reasonable weight. We are indeed called to self-discipline, for we are soldiers—soldiers of the Cross of Calvary.

Before I leave this field, I should like to give my personal opinion about anti-obesity medication, medication meant to help reduce weight. I must stress that the optimal method of weight reduction is through a healthy or proper diet and regular exercise.

In my opinion anti-obesity medication should be reserved for those who have health problems relating to their obesity, for example high blood pressure, diabetes, etc. It could also be used as an initial help for individuals very determined to lose weight through diet and exercise. They should be discontinued after a while, after they have served their initial purpose whilst the affected person maintains the habit of eating a healthy diet and engaging in regular exercise. That, however, is my personal view on the matter. One is free to accept or reject it.

My opinion is based on my experience in general practice. There have been instances in the past when some of my patients bent on reducing weight have requested me to prescribe them such medication. After the initial weight reduction, brought about not only by the medication, but also by their determination to maintain a healthy diet and engage in regular exercise, some came back a few weeks later to confess that while indeed the "soul was willing, the flesh was weak." That became evident after taking their respective weights. After the initial weight reduction in the few days following the beginning of the anti-obesity therapy, some had returned to their initial weights; some had even surpassed their pre-therapy weights.

Finally: it should be borne in mind that like almost every medication, anti-obesity drugs are not devoid of side effects.

On the matter of "good" and "bad" Cholesterol

Still on the measures that we can take to prevent disease, I want to touch briefly on cholesterol. The word *cholesterol* has gained a negative connotation over the last few years due partly to reports about it in the media. What many may not know is that it is needed for building and regulating cells. In other words, cholesterol is necessary for the normal functioning of our bodies. There are actually two types of cholesterol, low density lipoprotein (LDL) cholesterol as well as high density lipoprotein (HDL) cholesterol.

The negative effect of cholesterol on the body relates to LDL and not HDL. It is indeed true that too much LDL cholesterol in the body can cause problems to the affected person. This can lead to part of the LDL settling on the walls of the blood vessels to build up what is termed "plagues". In time, the lumen or the inner open space of the affected vessel can become narrower and narrower. This could eventually lead to the blockage of the vessel concerned. If this happens to the arteries supplying the heart and the brain, it could lead to a heart attack or stroke respectively.

It is important to reduce the amount of cholesterol consumed. One way of achieving this is to limit the consumption of food rich in cholesterol such as eggs, milk, cheese and meat.

HDL Cholesterol, in contrast to LDL Cholesterol, is known to have a beneficial effect on the vessels, preventing them from developing "plagues". Consequently HDL Cholesterol is sometimes referred to as "good" cholesterol.

Some foods such as olives, olive oil, and most nuts and nut oils (also known as monounsaturated fats) as well as vegetable oils play a beneficial role in the body by increasing HDL while at the same time lowering LDL.

It must however be borne in mind that about 75% of the body cholesterol is produced in the liver; therefore our diet alone is not the all-deciding factor in the level of cholesterol in our body.

Some individuals are also born with a genetic disorder known as Familial hypercholesterolemia. The body of the affected individual is not able to remove low density lipoprotein (LDL) cholesterol from the blood. This results in high levels of "bad" (LDL) Cholesterol in the blood of the affected person. This in turn can lead to the following symptoms, even at a young age:

- Fatty skin deposits (xanthomas) over the elbows, knees, buttocks, the cornea (white part of the eye), etc.
- Deposits of cholesterol in the eyelids (xanthelasmas).
- Arteriosclerosis (narrowing of the arteries).

KEEPING FIT THROUGH EXERCISE

What you are about to read as my introduction to the health benefits of exercise to the body has no pure scientific basis; it is, instead, based on my own observation.

It is no secret that despite the very difficult living conditions that prevail in several areas of the developing world, my native Ghana being an example, some individuals living there manage to make it past 80 years and beyond.

Obviously, several factors come into play concerning the longevity of an individual's life. Take, for instance, the case of my father who, despite the difficult living conditions he has been subjected to in our little village Mpintimpi, has made it to almost 90 years. How active one is in life, without doubt, counts as an important factor.

Indeed, during his young years, father was literally almost always on his feet during most of the day—walking to his farm, clearing virgin forests and felling huge trees with the aid of only an axe to prepare the land for cultivation, planting seeds in the cultivated land, weeding under his cocoa farm, and carrying loads on his head back home after a strenuous day's work on the farm. His daily activity did not end with his work on the farm. Back home he continued to be active in various other ways. As I mentioned earlier, his active life alone would not account for his longevity. Without doubt, however, it has contributed towards it.

There is indeed a general consensus among health care professionals concerning the beneficial effect of regular physical exercise to our health. Apart from preventing us from becoming overweight or obese, regular exercise can indeed help protect us from several diseases. These include heart disease, stroke, high blood pressure, Type 2 diabetes, obesity, back pain, and osteoporosis (a disease in which the bones become extremely porous and are subject to break or fracture). For some, exercise even helps to improve their mood.

There is clearly, therefore, a need for us to exercise our body on a regular basis. The question that arises is: how much exercise is enough? There is no clear-cut answer to the question. I will call for a common-sense approach. Much us we are called upon not to overeat, I think when it comes to exercise it is also important that we do not overdo it, that we do not do more than our body can cope with.

For example, if you have been inactive for a while it is better to start with less strenuous activities such as walking or swimming at a comfortable pace. Beginning at a slow pace will allow you to become physically fit without straining your body. Once you are in better shape, you can gradually do more strenuous activities.

Most experts agree that moderate exercise for 30 minutes every other day is adequate to help improve the cardiovascular function, to lose weight, reduce stress as well as lower cholesterol and blood pressure.

DO NOT "BURN-OUT" YOURSELF

We should not lead an idle life, not sit down doing nothing and hope that manna will fall from heaven to feed us. The Bible tells the story of how Almighty God fed the Israelites with manna in the wilderness. Today, we are called upon to co-operate with Almighty God, not only to feed ourselves but also to provide for our livelihood during our sojourn on planet earth.

Go to the ant, thou sluggard; consider her ways, and be wise: Which having no guide, overseer, or ruler, Provideth her meat in the summer, and gathereth her food in the harvest. How long wilt thou sleep, O sluggard? when wilt thou arise out of thy sleep? Yet a little sleep, a little slumber, a little folding of the hands to sleep:

So shall thy poverty come as one that travelleth, and thy want as an armed man. Proverbs 6: 6-11

God indeed helps those who help themselves. Still, it is important that we guard against overstraining or overworking ourselves. It could among other things, lead to what the doctors call Burn-Out Syndrome (defined as chronic work-related stress) which in turn could adversely affect our immune system.

I have heard the story of some citizens from my native Ghana resident in London who leave home in the morning to work eight hours at Workplace A, move on from there to Workplace B to do another six hours of work only to move to Workplace C to do another four hours of work.

Some hardly make it back home to have a shower before moving back to start another day's work at Workplace A. Where do they keep and change their clothing? Well, the story goes that some keep their toiletries in their bags. They have their showers at their places of work! As far as food is concerned, they either carry it along or purchase some from one of the numerous fast food chains around. And what about sleep? Well, according to the story, they do so during their travels on public transport—the Underground and the London buses. Some are said to fall so deep asleep during their journeys that they miss their stations and are usually awakened at the end station by the station assistants during their routine checks on the trains.

That kind of work ethic, I dare speculate, is not what King Solomon had in mind when he wrote his inspired words in Proverbs 6: 6-11!

The body of the individual I referred to may perhaps be able to cope with that degree of stress for a while. One does not need to have a degree in medical science or be a prophet, to predict that should that strain on the body continue for a while, it will sooner, rather than later lead to the breakdown of the individual involved. We are human beings after all, we are not machines. And even machines need periods of respite for maintenance and repair. The body can cope with stress over short periods, but stress, when it becomes chronic, can adversely affect our health and lead to the following: weakening of the immune system, headache, upset stomach, stomach ulcer, high blood pressure, heart attack, etc.

BREASTFEEDING AS A WAY OF DISEASE PREVENTION

Before I leave this section on the prevention of disease I want to touch on the issue of breastfeeding. Breastfeeding indeed belongs to the area of disease prevention, for apart from providing the means of energy and growth for the new-born, it also provides needed antibodies to boost the immune system of the new-born.

You and I are aware that today, industry has come up with formula milk. Now I am not saying that this is not a good thing. As in all instances of our existence, industry, once it has come up with a product, will go to great lengths to sort of push the product onto the consumer.

Agreed, there are instances when mothers are unable to breastfeed on health grounds. I should like at this stage to recall my childhood in my little village in Ghana. I remember at the time when I was growing up there when mainly as a result of disease a new mother was not able to breastfeed her baby, other women, those already nursing their babies, stepped in to help out. In some instances, some women who were even not breastfeeding at that time took over that function. Somehow the body registered the need to produce milk in the extraordinary circumstance and began producing milk!

As a Christian doctor, I want to appeal to my readers, my sisters in Christ, to, as far as possible, breastfeed their babies for a minimum of six months, due to the factors outlined below:

Protection against infection and diseases. As I mentioned above, breast milk is rich in antibodies. These are passed on to the child. This leads to a strengthening of the body's defence force. This helps to protect against some of the infections common in the early stage of life.

Antibodies passed from a nursing mother to her baby can help lower the occurrence of many conditions, including:

- ear infections
- diarrhoea
- respiratory infections
- meningitis

It has been established that breast-fed infants are less prone to diseases as compared to infants who receive formula.

Mothers living in a place like my little village Mpintimpi will tell you, usually during the time when they are breastfeeding their children, the children usually look well-nourished and also less susceptible to infections. The problem begins during the transition to normal feeding and thereafter. Soon they not only begin to display signs of malnutrition, they also become susceptible to infections.

Besides protecting against infections, the strengthening of the immune system can protect the baby against allergies which in turn could minimise the risk of developing asthma.

Nutrition and ease of digestion. As I mentioned earlier, the body requires carbohydrates, fat and protein to grow. All the three components are present in breast milk. The good thing for the baby is that they are present in a form that makes it easy for the new-born's immature digestive system to absorb them.

It's Free. Breast milk doesn't cost anything, so it is affordable to even the poorest mother walking the earth's surface. The author of these lines really does wonder what would have happened to him if his impoverished parents were forced to resort to formula milk to feed him!

Different tastes. It has been established that breast milk has different flavours depending on the meals eaten by the mother. Breastfed babies are thus introduced to different tastes through their mothers' breast milk.

Ease of Availability. It's available whenever and wherever the baby needs to be fed. Mothers who breastfeed are thus spared the last-minute dashes to the store for more formula as well as the need to warm up bottles, sometimes in the middle of the night.

Breastfeeding mothers are able to actively go about their activities with their babies, knowing that they'll have food available whenever their little one is hungry.

Obesity prevention. Some studies have found that breastfeeding may help prevent obesity.

Skin-to-skin. The skin-to-skin contact between mother and child in breastfeeding can enhance the emotional connection between mother and infant.

Breastfeeding does not only facilitate the health of the baby, but that of the mother as well. Breastfeeding helps burn the calories of the mother and helps shrink the uterus, so nursing mothers are able to return to their pre-pregnancy shape and weight a lot sooner than those who resort to formula.

Studies have also shown that breastfeeding helps lower the risk of contracting cancer of the breast, the ovary and the womb.

PART 2

TERMINOLOGY DEFINED

B efore I tackle some of the most common diseases around, I shall spend some time to explain some of the common terminologies that may confront us not only in this book, but in our day-to-day involvement with issues relating to our health. These are:

- The Immune System
- Infection
- Fever
- DNA and Genes.

Chapter 3

The Immune System

⌒⌒

There are millions upon millions of microscopic organisms all over the place poised to attack our bodies, to cause harm to us.

Someone might ask, "Why did a loving God expose us to such organisms in the first place?"

I really do not want to answer that question. How can I, mortal that I am, read the mind of the Almighty God? Still, I dare make an attempt to answer the question, at least based on the limited understanding placed at my disposal by Almighty God. I want to stress—my explanation is based on my own insight into the matter. You are free to accept or reject it.

Yes, I do sincerely believe that when God Almighty first created Adam and Eve, there was no need for such a defence system. Yes, I do believe that prior to the fall of Humanity, Adam and Eve lived in harmony not only with the macroscopic but also with the microscopic world. As a result, there was no need for a defence shield.

With the curse came human suffering and, worst of all, death. All of a sudden not only did the macroscopic world become our enemies but also the microscopic.

Even then, God Almighty did not leave us alone, but rather put into place in our bodies a defence system to help us cope with the hazards we would be exposed to in life.

Our immune system is not only intelligent; it is complex and at the same time sophisticated. I do not want to delve into details in the matter. Those interested to know more are advised to source the relevant literature on the topic. What we have to know is that we can through our attitude, diet, lifestyle, etc., either strengthen or weaken the defensive capabilities of our formidable army.

Chapter 4

Infection

∞

Infection is a term we all encounter on a regular basis. What does it mean?

I will try to explain it from a Christian perspective, for one of the arguments brought up by those who do not believe in God, or those who are angry with Him, is: if God is love, why then did He create the bacteria, the viruses, indeed, the parasites to trouble us and threaten our lives?

As I mentioned earlier, I believe, as recorded in the Bible, that at the very beginning when Almighty God created the heavens and the earth, everything was good and perfect. The micro- as well as the macro-organisms lived in harmony with one another.

After the Fall of Mankind, the harmony was disturbed. Instead of living in harmony with each other, created beings began to pester one another.

In the case of natural enemies such as the lion, the tiger, the snake, we are able to see them. We can, as a result, attempt to flee them long before they make an attempt to get at us.

That, however, is not the case when it comes to micro-organisms—they are invisible to our naked eye and so we are incapable of fleeing from them. Examples of the microscopic organisms are bacteria, viruses, yeast, fungi, etc.

As I mentioned above, the Lord has given our bodies a defence system, the immune system, to help fight the attacking organisms. Sometimes, however, these enemy organisms are able to overcome our defence system (we saw earlier on how our own attitude can contribute to the weakening of our defence system), which can lead to one of several infectious diseases.

In Ephesians 6:12 we read:

For we wrestle not against flesh and blood, but against principalities, against powers, against the rulers of the darkness of this world, against spiritual wickedness in high places.

Well, we fight not only against principalities and spiritual wickedness in high places, but also against hordes of invisible micro-organisms poised on attacking and harming us.

Diseases brought about by such micro-organisms are classified as infectious diseases.

The list of infectious diseases is long. They range from the common cold to the potentially life-threatening diseases like cholera, malaria, meningitis, etc.

Infectious diseases can be passed on from one person to another. There are several avenues by which this can happen:

- Droplets: Infectious organisms may be passed on by means of droplets containing them. This can happen through sneezing, coughing, talking, etc.
- Ingestion: This can be achieved through eating contaminated food or drinking contaminated water.
- Sexual Contact. As I mentioned earlier, several kinds of infection can be sexually transmitted.
- Skin: Infectious organisms can penetrate the body following injury to the skin.

Chapter 5

Fever

∞

W hen I worked as a family doctor in Dusseldorf in Germany, the majority of my patients were from Ghana.

On not a few occasions some of them came to the consulting room with the words, "Doc, please help me—I have fever."

In most instances the temperature of the patient turned out to be normal.

Thereupon, I made it clear to the patient that he or she had no fever.

"But I feel feverish, Doc. I really do believe I have fever!"

It is indeed important for a doctor to understand the cultural background of the patients he or she is dealing with to properly understand their needs! Whereas a patient from Ghana will tell you "I have fever" when he/she wants to let you know he/she feels generally unwell, an English patient will tell you he/she is "feeling poorly". Indeed, prior to my arrival in the UK it never occurred to me that a person who was vomiting would describe that condition as *"I am being sick."*

This leads me to the term fever as it is applied in medicine. To help us maintain a stable milieu within our body sys tem in the presence of ever-changing environmental conditions, Almighty God put into place in our bodies several self-regulatory mechanisms. This is particularly important, since our body was created to function within an almost constant body temperature range of between 36.5–37.5 °C (98–100 °F).

How do they do so on a planet that can be as hot as the Sahara and as cold as the Arctic?

Well, the hypothalamus, an area in our brain, is assigned the responsibility of maintaining a normal temperature range as stated above.

The hypothalamus is responsible not only for the maintenance of a constant body temperature but several other regulatory functions in the body. The hypothalamus achieves this goal with the help of agents known as thermo receptors located in several parts of the body.

Disease, in particular, infectious disease, can disturb this control mechanism and lead to a rise in body temperature above the set norm. A fever can be caused by many different conditions ranging from benign to potentially serious.

Moderate rises in body temperature do not usually require treatment, for the body is capable of coping with such rises.

Whatever the cause of fever, the moment it rises beyond a certain point, especially in children, there is a need to take steps to help bring it down. Though the underlying cause may not cause problems, the very fact that the temperature has risen above a certain level could lead to problems including what is known as febrile convulsion.

This takes me back again to my childhood days. Malaria was and is still endemic in Ghana. I remember in not rare instances, little children whose bodies had turned "hot", as we put it, who would suddenly begin to have a fit. Lay people as we were in the matters of medicine, we at that juncture instinctively began to pour cold water on the affected child. In many instances that led to an improvement of the condition. We did not really understand the mechanism involved. Naturally we were delighted at the favourable outcome of our action. If only we had known that the rising temperature could lead to the fit, we would have administered paracetamol (if indeed it was available) earlier on to avert the situation.

Chapter 6

Blame the Naughty Genes!

∞

I n this chapter, I will briefly explain the terms DNA and genes. They may not affect you directly. Still, I think it is important that you get at least some idea about them, for these days one hears and reads a lot about them. DNA stands for desoxyribonucleicacid (**D**esoxyribo**N**ucleic**A**cid).

What then is DNA? I will offer an explanation from a Christian perspective.

The Bible states that in the beginning God created all living things, including Human Beings. He empowered us with the ability to reproduce and multiply. The information needed to do so was encoded on a microscopic particle that has come to be known as DNA.

It is important to stress that DNA was created by Almighty God and not invented by anyone. It is not like the telephone or the electric bulb or the printing machine that was conceived by the brain of a human being. When it comes to DNA the best we can boast about is that we discovered it in the cell, studied it and came to understand how it works.

As at November 2010, the population of the world is said to be around 6.8 billion individuals. Now, apart from identical twins, each and every one of us has a unique DNA. That is what makes us look different from each other. Now, those who say there is no God, in my opinion, must be credited with incredible faith, to hold on to their conviction. That in my opinion is what is preventing them from recognising the awesomeness of the Power behind the universe—the power that could store information on a microscopic particle that is so unique as to be able to form each and every one of 6.7 billion individuals (identical twins excluded) walking the surface of the earth *differently*. I am humbled, immensely humbled, by the power and authority of the LIVING GOD—indeed I am, to the very bottom of my heart!

Now let us consider the gene. For the layman, things can be confusing in regard to the DNA and the gene. Even the author, who has done his "apprenticeship" with the medical scientist, it is not always easy to figure out the relationship between DNA, Genes, Chromosomes and several other issues related to the cell. Doesn't that also point to the ingenuity of He who put them in place to start with?

To help you understand the concept of a gene, I shall consider the game of football, also known as soccer.

A football team consists of 11 players, each having a different role. We can think of the whole team of 11 players as DNA, with the genes being the individual players. The "goalkeeper gene" has the duty of keeping the goal; the "attacker gene" has to keep on scoring goals, otherwise their team faces the danger of relegation from the English Premier league; the "defender gene" has to defend well, otherwise their opponents could humiliate them with a goal harvest. Indeed, all the 11 genes that make up the DNA Football team should perform well to ensure the wellbeing of the whole team.

That is not usually the case. In real life a football player may suffer broken jaws, broken teeth, a strained leg causing him to limp, etc. A football player who has suffered a broken limb can, under normal circumstances, give birth to a normal child—a child who will not be born with a broken limb just because his dad had a broken limb at the time he impregnated his mother.

That is where the difference arises between players of the DNA football team and the real DNA genes. In the case of the latter, they can indeed pass on their defects to the offspring of the affected individual.

That could then lead to what is termed "genetically transmitted diseases". For example, a parent suffering from sickle cell, which is caused by a defect in a gene, can pass this on to his or her offspring.

The illustration may not be perfect, but I hope it is enough to permit you to understand when, later in the book, I say something like "sickle cell anaemia is a genetically transmitted disease".

Now before I leave the country of the DNA and Genes, I shall pass a comment. I have the impression that these days the scientific world is seeking to trace everything that goes on in our lives, including even our moral shortcomings, to our genes. If we cannot control our appetite for food, it is "in our genes"; if we are attracted to a person of the same sex it is attributed to our genes; if we over indulge in drink and allow Monster Alcohol to control our brains, it is still the fault of our dubious genes!

It won't really surprise me if a time comes in the future when we shut the doors to all our courtrooms and send our judges, magistrates, solicitors and court clerks home to rest for ever. The reason? Our naughty genes having completely taken control of us, and no one will evermore be legally held accountable for any shortcomings, criminal, moral or what have you.

PART 3

COMMON MEDICAL CONDITIONS TREATED

∽

A s my German driving teacher taught us from the outset, when we are in traffic, there are certain factors that could affect us that we have no control over. The same applies to the matter of our health. No matter what preventive measures we adopt, we can still fall victim to disease. It is therefore important that we keep ourselves informed about some of the common diseases that afflict mankind. Understanding what causes them and the symptoms to look out for will enable us to recognise them, preferably in their early stages. Apart from primary prevention, early recognition and treatment forms another important aspect in the fight against disease. This is particularly true in the case of cancer.

I will therefore turn my attention to some of the common conditions that afflict us. I will in most cases observe the following pattern:

1) Cause: I will explain the cause of disease based on the latest knowledge available to medical science.
2) Symptoms: I will highlight the common symptoms associated with the condition.
3) Risk factors.
4) Diagnosis.

5) Treatment: I will highlight the treatment possibilities. Even though I will not mention prayer as a part of the therapy in all instances, I do believe that prayer is a powerful weapon in every stage of the battle against disease.

Is any sick among you? let him call for the elders of the church; and let them pray over him, anointing him with oil in the name of the Lord: And the prayer of faith shall save the sick, and the Lord shall raise him up; and if he have committed sins, they shall be forgiven him. James 5:14-15

Chapter 7

Headache

I think it is superfluous to attempt to define the term headache; everyone has in his or her lifetime experienced this condition.
Medical science knows two types of headache.

- **Primary Headache:** This type of headache stands on its own. In other words it is not related to any kind of disease.
- **Secondary Headache:** This is the headache that happens when the patient is afflicted by another disease. For example, one of the symptoms of the common flu is a headache. In other words, the headache is secondary to the flu infection. Sometimes, however, a headache may be the symptom of a more serious condition or disease, such as a brain tumour or meningitis. Other examples of medical conditions that can lead to headache are high blood pressure, dental abscess, eye conditions, etc.

PRIMARY HEADACHE

Unlike the secondary headache, primary headaches are not caused by another disease or condition. The three common types of primary headache are: tension headache, migraine and cluster headaches.

- **Tension Headache:** Each and every one of us might have experienced a tension headache at one stage in our life. It is characterised by a dull, steady and achy pain on both sides of the head. The pain usually begins gradually and increases over a period of time. Tension headaches are associated with stress, anxiety and depression.
- **Migraine:** This is an intense, throbbing, pounding or pulsating pain that is often experienced on one side of the head. Victims of the disease usually report experiencing symptoms that serve as a harbinger or foreteller that announces the onset of their pain. These include visual disturbances such as light flashing before the eyes, a funny taste in the mouth or a strange smell.
- **Cluster Headaches:** These are a type of headache similar to migraine and sometimes described as agonising or excruciating by the affected person. Victims may also experience severe pain in the eye or temple on one side of the head as well as a watering of the eye and a runny nose. Cluster headaches may be triggered by certain kinds of drugs and also by alcohol.

DIAGNOSIS

- Taking the patient's history, including family history (it has been observed that some families are prone to headaches such as migraines).
- X-ray: Though it may not be useful in certain cases, in the case of a brain tumour, X-ray can be a helpful tool in the diagnosis.
- CT & MRI-Scan: These can help reveal several causes of secondary headache such as brain tumours, cysts, abscesses, aneurysm etc.

THERAPY

At the time I was growing up in my little village, though we could not count ourselves with the most sophisticated of people, we were nevertheless aware that Paracetamol, Aspirin and APC (which stands for aspirin, paracetamol and codeine) could help relieve headache. So whenever any of us was afflicted with the condition, we made our way to one of the few petty traders in the village selling them (they were usually sold as single tablets!), bought a few, took them and hoped for a favourable outcome.

Indeed, common primary headaches respond well to the above-named medication. We should however guard against overusing them. Failure to do so could lead to a paradox situation in which the analgesics or painkillers that are supposed to cure our headaches themselves become their cause. Indeed, overuse of such tablets could themselves lead to headaches—rebound or analgesic headaches, as they are called.

Chapter 8

Anaemia

The term *anaemia* refers to the situation when there is less than the normal number of red blood cells or less than the normal quantity of haemoglobin in the blood. Haemoglobin is a pigment found in the red blood cell. It has the primary function of transporting oxygen from the lungs to the body tissues. Indeed, it is the pigment haemoglobin that gives red blood cells their characteristic red colour. When there is a shortage of either the red blood cells or haemoglobin or both, the capacity of the blood to transport oxygen round the body is decreased.

To understand the effect of anaemia to the body, it is important to understand the role blood plays in the body. These are the following:

1. It transports oxygen away from the lungs and around the body; and carbon dioxide from the cells back to the lungs to be breathed away.
2. It transports nutrients to the cells.
3. It carries waste products away from the cells to organs such as the kidney and liver for excretion from the body.
4. It helps the body maintain a constant temperature.
5. With the help of the white blood cells, it helps to defend the body from various organisms that invade the body to cause harm to it.

6. Blood also carries substances that help blood to clot in case of injury and in so doing help prevent blood loss.

Blood has two components: the liquid part, also known as plasma, and the cells floating in it. Dissolved in the plasma are various substances including electrolytes, nutrients, vitamins, hormones, clotting factors, and infection-fighting antibodies.

The cellular part of blood is about ninety-nine per cent red blood cells; the remaining one per cent is white blood cells.

The adult human body contains approximately five litres of blood; it makes up seven to eight per cent of a person's body weight.

TYPES OF ANAEMIA

There are three main types of anaemia:

1) Anaemia caused by increased red cell destruction, for example sickle cell anaemia.
2) Anaemia caused by decreased red cell formation. This can result from the following: poor diet, diet deficient in folic acid, iron and Vitamin B12; chronic disease such as HIV/Aids; Cancer, etc.
3) Anaemia resulting from blood loss: injury to the body, diseases that cause profuse bleeding and heavy menstrual bleeding could also lead to anaemia.

SIGNS AND SYMPTOMS OF ANAEMIA

These include the following:

1) Fatigue (feeling tired all the time)
2) Headache
3) Dizzy spells

4) Shortness of breadth
5) Palpitations (rapid and irregular heartbeat)

TREATMENT

Treatment of anaemia aims at correcting the underlying cause of the condition with the end goal of either increasing the number of red blood cells in the body or the amount of haemoglobin carried by the red blood cells, or both.

For example:

- Iron-Deficiency anaemia is treated with iron tablets or in some cases injections.
- Vitamin supplements may be taken to replace folic acid and vitamin B12 in people with poor eating habits.
- Some people suffer from what is known as pernicious anaemia. In such individuals, their digestive system is incapable of absorbing sufficient amounts of vitamin B12 in their meal. Such individuals are treated with monthly injections of vitamin B12.
- If anaemia is caused by chronic or severe disease, treatment of the underlying cause could lead to a normalisation of the condition.
- In certain instances, blood transfusion could become necessary to correct anaemia.

SICKLE CELL ANAEMIA

Before I leave the area of anaemia, I shall devote some lines to the condition known as sickle cell anaemia.

What does the term stand for?

Medical science refers to normal haemoglobin as HbA. Each individual is endowed with two copies of the haemoglobin gene. A completely healthy individual thus carries two HbAs—one from each parent.

People with sickle cell anaemia have a type of haemoglobin known as sickle haemoglobin (HbS), which is different from normal haemoglobin (HbA).

Those who have one HbA gene and one HbS gene are said to have sickle cell trait and are referred to as carriers. Those with sickle cell anaemia have two HbS genes

The red blood cells of a person suffering from full-blown sickle cell anaemia are destroyed faster than would be the case of the person carrying normal red blood cells. Sickle red blood cells have a life-span of approximately ten to twenty days compared to that of normal cells, which is between eighty and one hundred and twenty days. The end result of the above situation is that the individual born with the condition has to live with chronic anaemia.

Normal red blood cells are smooth, round, and quite flexible. As a result they can bend and flex easily, and so travel around the blood vessels easily. Sickle cells on their part are stiff and sticky and as a result are not able to move easily through blood vessels. Furthermore, they tend to form clumps and get stuck in smaller blood vessels. This leads in the end to the blockage of the small blood vessels of the affected person which in turn leads to the disruption of blood circulation to the end organ.

SYMPTOM

- **Sickle Cell Crisis:** Blockage of a blood vessel causes an attack known as a crisis. This is more likely to happen when the person is stressed by another illness, exhaustion, cold, dehydration, low oxygen levels (such as living in high altitudes or flying).
- **Organ Damage**: The intermittent disruption of blood flow brought about by blocked vessels can lead to damage of organs such as the liver, kidney, lungs, heart and spleen.
- **Chronic Pain:** The blockage of the vessels can also lead to severe recurring pain, especially in the bones.
- **Anaemia:** The constant breakdown of the red blood cells leads to anaemia.

- **Chronic Infection**: Sickle cell anaemia is also associated with recurring infections.

TREATMENT

There's no cure for sickle cell anaemia, but the frequency and severity of crises and their complications can be reduced by avoiding the triggers and prompt recognition and treatment of a crisis.

One can take measures to minimise the effect.

These include:

- Eating a good diet and taking supplements of folic acid, vitamin D and zinc.
- Avoiding smoking and alcohol (both of which can affect the condition of blood vessels).
- Vaccination against infections such as the flu, pneumococcus meningitis and Hepatitis B, etc. will all help reduce the risk of a crisis. Some patients are given long term antibiotics.
- Avoiding dehydration, cold temperatures as well as overexertion.
- In some instances, patients are given long term antibiotics.

TRANSMISSION OF SICKLE CELL

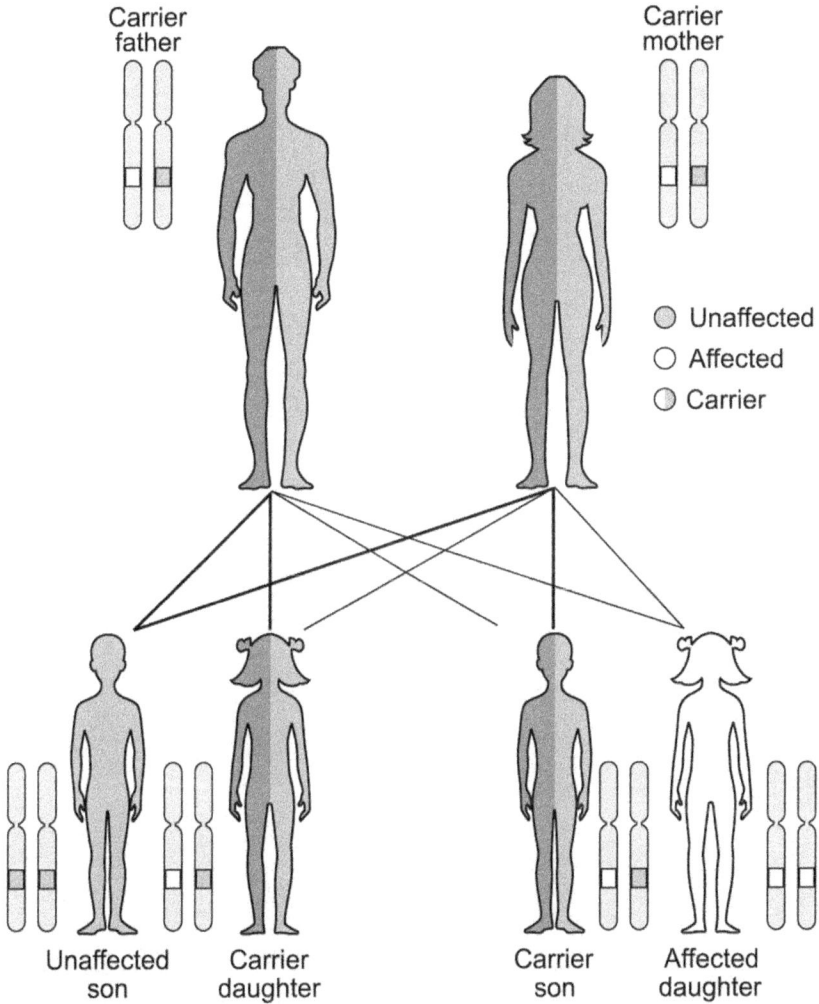

Illustration of how sickle cell is genetically transmitted

PREVETION

Sickle cell anaemia can only occur when two people who carry the sickle cell trait have a child together. It is therefore advisable for an individual who is a carrier to avoid marrying another carrier of the disease... easier said than done! In the real world, who would go around testing the genetic constitution of a person he or she is attracted to before falling in love with such an individual?

Chapter 9

Hernia

When I was growing up in my little village, there was a resident who had developed a hydrocele of the scrotum, a medical condition that leads to the accumulation of fluid in the scrotum. In the individual in question, the hydrocele had attained, without exaggeration, a really monstrous dimension. Those who are strange to the environment in which I grew up might ask: "Why didn't he seek medical attention?" The answer in short is poverty, poverty, poverty.

In the course of time word began to spread in the little settlement to the effect that one of the residents had been diagnosed with inguinal hernia.

The doctors had recommended surgery. He had begged them to allow him to return to the village to gather the needed financial resources. Partly because he had in the meantime been feeling better, partly because he could not come up with the money required, he refused to return to the hospital.

In the course of time someone told me that as much as the huge hydrocele of our co-resident was without doubt an embarrassment to him, it was not life threatening. On the other hand another resident afflicted with a hernia had a more dangerous condition that could kill him.

You may call it health education "Mpintimpi style". The doctors and other health professionals among us, those conversant with both conditions, will agree that my "health education instructor" was after all not entirely wrong in his assertion, for indeed a hernia can become life-threatening whereas a hydrocele of the scrotum rarely will.

WHAT IS HERNIA?

Our internal organs are wrapped in a transparent membrane (a plastic-like sac) called the peritoneum; this sack in turn is protected by the muscles of the stomach wall. The abdominal wall thus acts as a protective cover for our internal organs, in particular our intestines.

In some instances, a tear occurs in the protecting wall. When this happens, parts of the internal organs, especially the intestines, bulge through the tear and appear as a lump under the skin. This is what is referred to as a hernia. Sometimes the weakness is already present in children, for example around the navel (umbilical hernia).

This again brings back memories of the time when I was growing up in my little village. There were a few of my peers walking around, clothed only in children slips, displaying what is known in my native Twi language as *funuma purudu*. The term stands literally for a protruding navel. Some of the navel hernias had indeed attained considerable sizes. Innocent as we were as regards the cause and also the potential life threatening complications of strangulation, we used to taunt them, indeed make fun of them.

Apart from the navel, the groin is another common hernia site.

When a hernia first occurs the affected person may have a feeling that something has given way and may experience a little pain. The pain soon wears off. Later, a lump appears. This doesn't hurt and may get bigger on coughing.

The lump may from time to time disappear only to reappear again (as the herniating tissue slips back into place and then protrudes again.)

In most cases hernias just cause discomfort and are a bit of a nuisance. The real worry with hernias is that they may strangulate. Put another way, they could become stuck in the weak point in the muscles which in turn could lead to an interruption in its blood supply.

Without an emergency operation to release it and restore its blood supply, some of the tissue could die, leading to serious illness. As I was taught by the "medical experts" in my little village, it could lead to death.

RISK FACTORS

Following are some of the risk factors for the development of hernia.

- **Gender:** Men are particularly disposed to experience hernia of the groin because of their anatomy. (I shall not delve into further details.)
- **Inter-abdominal pressure:** Any activity that leads to a rise in the pressure within the abdomen such as lifting heavy objects, coughing, even straining on the toilet, can cause a weakness or tear in the abdominal wall, or force intestinal contents out through a weakness.
- **Previous surgery:** Surgery on the abdominal wall creates a vulnerable spot, which can later lead to a hernia. This type of hernia is also referred to as incisional hernia.

TREATMENT

Treatment usually involves surgery. Surgery may be through the traditional method of cutting and repair or by way of the so-called pin-hole surgery.

Chapter 10

High Blood Pressure

∞

One day several relations of Rita, my wife, paid us a visit. In the course of the interaction one of our guests spotted the blood pressure measuring machine in the living room.

"Doc, can you please measure my blood pressure? I do not remember the last time I had it checked."

"No problem!" I replied. Without delay, I went into action to measure it. It read 115 over 70.

"Normal; no cause for concern!" I told him.

"Would you mind checking mine as well!" his other half requested.

"Of course not!" Like her husband, her pressure was also okay.

Soon it turned out to be a kind of "children's game", for everyone present wanted to have his or her blood pressure checked!

Soon I would become not only a messenger of good news, but also of news not so pleasant—for, as it turned out, the blood pressure of one of our visitors was extremely high, requiring treatment as early as practicable!

Our visitor knew all along that his wife's blood pressure was high, a fact that had required her to take medication. What he was not aware of, however, was the fact that he had also developed the condition. (That is not to say that his wife had passed it on to him. No, high blood pressure is not, as it were, an infectious disease that our spouses or our neighbours can pass on to us. As we shall soon find out, we may inherit it from our parents, but that is as far as it goes.)

As it turned out, our relation had been living with high blood pressure, a veritable "time bomb", as it were, without being aware of it! That indeed is one of the disturbing aspects of high blood pressure.

If you and I visit a restaurant and eat food infested with the salmonella bacteria, our respective bodies would likely react in a matter of hours with nausea, vomiting and in some cases diarrhoea. Soon it would become clear to you and me that something is wrong with our body system. We would then take appropriate steps to reverse the situation.

The situation, unfortunately, is different, when it comes to high blood pressure. One may indeed live with it for a considerable period of time without knowing it!

Then, all of a sudden, one day, just like a time bomb waiting to explode, it does indeed burst out—sometimes in deep sleep. It could manifest itself as a stroke or a heart attack that could lead the individual never to awaken from sleep.

"He was fine, in real good spirits when he [or she] bade me goodnight!" the shattered spouse or relation might tell you.

If that individual happened to reside in my native Ghana, his or her relations would, with all likelihood, blame witchcraft, wizards, jujumen, etc., for having cut short the life of the successful businessman or woman.

Indeed, the only way for a person to know whether he/she lives with the condition of high blood pressure is to have the pressure checked by a competent person—a health assistant, a nurse, a doctor, etc. Having said that by way of introduction, I shall give a brief overview of the condition.

Almighty God placed blood into the body system to help transport oxygen and nutrients to various parts of the body. On its journey back to the heart, it picks up the waste products of metabolism for further transport to the lungs, the liver, the kidney etc.

Almighty God placed the heart, an amazing muscular pump, in the chest to pump blood around the body. In order for the blood to be pumped around the body, pressure must be generated by the heart.

Medical science uses the term *hypertension* when blood is forced through the arteries with an increased force.

Blood pressure is expressed as two numbers, for example "120 over 80".

The top number is known as the systolic pressure. This stands for the pressure generated by the heart on beating.

The bottom number, known as the diastolic pressure, stands for the pressure in the circulatory system when the heart is resting between beats.

A person's blood pressure is generally considered normal if it stays slightly above or below 120/80. A person whose systolic blood pressure is consistently 140 or higher or whose diastolic pressure is 90 or higher is generally considered to have high blood pressure.

CAUSES

In about 90% of cases, medical science has not found any reason to explain why someone's blood pressure is high. This condition is known as essential or primary hypertension.

In the remaining 10 per cent of cases, there is an underlying cause. This is called secondary hypertension.

Some of the main causes for secondary hypertension are:

- chronic kidney diseases
- diseases in the arteries supplying the kidneys
- chronic alcohol abuse
- hormonal disturbances
- endocrine tumours

SYMPTOMS

As the example I cited at the beginning demonstrates, initially high blood pressure may not cause symptoms and go unnoticed until it leads to complications such as a stroke or heart attack.

In severe cases of the condition, some of the following symptoms could become apparent:

- headache
- sleepiness
- confusion
- coma

RISK FACTORS

Medical science has identified the following risks factors for the development of high blood pressure:

- Family Background: The condition tends to occur in families. For example, if your father or mother has the condition, you are also at the risk of developing it as well.
- Obesity/Overweight: It has been established that people who are obese or overweight have a high risk of developing high blood pressure.
- Smoking: Apart from the more common risk factors associated with it such as lung cancer and other respiratory diseases, smoking has also been identified as a risk factor for the development of high blood pressure.
- Diabetes: Diabetes itself does not lead to high blood pressure. However, it has been established that the two conditions tend to occur together in the same individual.
- Kidney Disease: Certain types of kidney diseases lead the afflicted person to develop a high blood pressure.

TREATMENT

I have outlined above the possible risk factors for the development of high blood pressure. Avoiding the risk factors could help prevent disease.

If, despite such measures, the blood pressure remains high, treatment with medication would become necessary.

Such medication would need to be taken regularly and in some cases for the rest of the individual's life. Talking of taking medication on a regular basis! As a GP I have to keep on reminding my patients to do exactly that. There are indeed some who, after the medication has led to a normalisation of the blood pressure, decide to stop taking it. This could eventually lead to a re-bound effect in which the pressure shoots up again.

MEDICATION

There are several medications in use. They are usually placed in groups. Examples of the groups of medication in use are as follows:

- ACE Inhibitors
- Angiotensin-II receptor antagonists
- Beta-Blockers
- Alpha-Blockers
- Calcium-Channel Blockers Diuretics

I shall not consider the groups in detail. You may consult your family doctor for further details.

***

LOW BLOOD PRESSURE

Before I leave the area relating to our blood pressure, I shall impart some information on low blood pressure. In considering the possible complications of high blood pressure vis-a-vis low blood pressure, I usually tell patients with low blood pressure to be, as it were, happy that they have a low rather than a high blood pressure.

In the case of low blood pressure, the heart is pumping blood at a pressure below the average expected of a normal human being.

Such individuals may feel dizzy and have the feeling that they might "pass out" especially on standing up. The reason behind this feeling may not be hard to figure out. The brain is very sensitive to oxygen and nutrients supplied by blood. When one stands up, the heart is required, at least momentarily, to pump blood with extra force in response to the altered position of the body. For the person with a low blood pressure the pressure generated by the heart may not be adequate.

Chapter 11

Heart Attack

∞

The human heart is indeed a masterpiece of God's creation. It begins its pumping activity early in an individual's development and works dutifully around the clock. It works during the day, as we go about life's activities, and at night when we are deep asleep; it works in our joys and in our sorrows; it works in toil and in ease; it works in the cold of the winter and the heat of summer. Indeed, no matter the time of day, the season of the year, or the state of our minds, this automatic pump Almighty God fixed into our chests keeps dutifully pumping day in and day out to sustain us.

Assuming an average pumping rate of seventy per minute, our heart pumps 100,800 times a day, or 36,792,000 times a year. In a life spanning seventy years, that amounts to approximately 2.3 billion times.

Like all other organs of the body, the human heart is not free from disease. This leads me to the term *heart attack* or *myocardial infarction*.

The heart muscles do not derive their blood supply directly from the blood being pumped from the heart's lumen or inner cavity. Instead, the blood supply to the muscles of the heart themselves is achieved by way of vessels known as the coronary arteries and their tributaries or branches. These are located on the outside walls of the heart.

As we might deduce from the above observations, the heart is a very busy muscular pump. As a result it needs a good supply of blood. Any interruption or blockage of the supply route of the coronary arteries may lead to the demise of the individual concerned.

A heart attack occurs when blood flow to part of the heart is blocked, often by a blood clot, causing damage to the affected muscle.

If the blood supply is cut off for a short time, the muscles may regain vitality. On the other hand if the blood supply is interrupted for a considerable period of time, it could lead to irreversible damage to the heart muscles. That in its turn could lead to the failure or the inability of the muscles to continue pumping blood. Depending on the extent of muscle damage, the situation could cause the heart to cease its pumping activity altogether, a situation which if not reversed within a short period of time, will lead to the death of the individual.

Heart Attack

RISK FACTORS

- **Smoking.** Smoking damages the interior walls of arteries including those supplying the heart. This favours the deposition of cholesterol and other substances on the walls of the vessels to form what is known as arteriosclerotic plagues. In time this could lead to a blockage of the vessel concerned.

- **High blood pressure.** Over time, high blood pressure can damage arteries, including those that supply the heart.
- **High blood cholesterol.** A high level of LDL ("bad") cholesterol, can favour the formation of arteriosclerotic plagues and in so doing lead to myocardial infarction or heart attack.
- **Family history of heart attack.** If your parents, grandparents or siblings have had heart attacks, you may be at risk, too. Your family may have a genetic condition that raises the risk of a heart attack.
- **Lack of physical activity.** Individuals who undertake regular exercise have a better cardiovascular fitness, which decreases their overall risk of heart attack. On the other hand, inactivity increases the risk of suffering a heart attack.
- **Obesity.** Being overweight raises the risk of heart disease because it is associated with high blood cholesterol levels, high blood pressure and diabetes.
- **Stress.** Studies have shown that those living a stressful lifestyle have an increased risk for developing a heart attack.

SYMPTOMS

Some symptoms associated with a heart attack are:

- Chest pain, usually a central, crushing pain, which may travel into the left arm or up into the neck or jaw, and persists for more than a few minutes. Unlike angina, the pain doesn't ease at rest. Sometimes the symptoms could be mild, which could be mistaken for indigestion.
- Shortness of breath or difficulty breathing.
- Sweating.
- Light-headedness.

- Dizziness.
- Palpitation.
- Nausea and vomiting.

TREATMENT

Heart attacks must be recognised and treated as quickly as possible because once a coronary artery is blocked, the heart muscle will die within four to six hours.

Signs to look out for in cardiac arrest

Before I leave the topic, I want to provide a brief overview of the measures that should be taken when we witness someone experiencing a cardiac arrest.

We should bear in mind that time is in the true sense of the word of the essence in such a situation. Each minute of delay reduces the chances of survival considerably.

Following are the signs to look out for in cardiac arrest:

- no palpable pulse.
- unconsciousness.
- apnoea (absence of breathing).

Emergency Measures in Cardiac Arrest

If available, call the emergency service. Whilst you wait you should undertake the emergency measure I am about to touch on. If, on the other hand, you happen to reside in a remote area such as Otwenbeweate in my native Ghana, calling the emergency service will be out of the question. As you undertake the measures outline below, your only other weapon will be prayer—yes, prayer to Almighty God for Divine intervention. That would be all that you could count on.

Immediate measures for resuscitation in cardiac arrest

1. Hold the patient and shake him or her from the shoulders.
2. Ask him loudly in the ear whether he can listen to you.
3. Open the airway by lifting the chin upwards; this will facilitate easy breathing of the patient.
4. Check whether the patient is breathing. Look for chest movements and feel the air from the mouth of the patient. If effective breathing is present, then lay the person in a straight line with tilted chin.
5. If breathing is slow and not spontaneous, begin artificial (mouth-to-mouth) respiration immediately. It is important to check pulse and heartbeat at short intervals.
6. If there are signs of circulation, continue the mouth-to-mouth breathing for a while until spontaneous breathing is established. In the meantime it is important to keep on checking circulation at short intervals.
7. If no circulation is present, then compress the chest at the rate of about 100 per minute. Care should be taken to make a proper effort at compression. This should be forceful enough but not violent as rib injury may take place in such an instance. The current recommended chest compression to rescue breaths is 30:2. In other words 30 rapid chest compressions should be followed by 2 rescue breaths. This is the case for adults.
8. In case of **infants and children**, the ratio is 15:2 cycles when **two** rescuers are involved. If it involves one rescuer the ratio is as in adults, that is, 30:2.

Chapter 12

Stroke

⌒⌒

The brain is the most complex organ in the body. It is divided into two sides, or hemispheres, each controlling the opposite side of the body and different areas of activity. The left hemisphere controls cognition (thinking) and language, plus movement and sensation on the right-hand side of the body. The right hemisphere controls functions involved in more visual-spatial skills, such as the ability to judge distances, size, form and where things are in space (which may affect skills such as map reading, for example), as well as movement and sensation on the left side of the body.

The brain regulates absolutely everything in the body—breathing, moving, sweating, sleeping, waking, feeling, thoughts, speech, etc. A constant supply of blood to deliver oxygen and nutrients to the brain cells is an essential pre-condition for the optimal function of the brain.

An interruption in the blood supply to the brain is termed a stroke. There are two types of stroke: ischaemic and haemorrhagic strokes.

- **Ischaemic stroke**. This is the more common of the two, accounting for around 80 per cent of all cases of stroke. This is the result of a blockage of one or more of the arteries supplying the brain with oxygenated blood, the blockage being caused by a blood clot.

Bleeding into the brain in hemorrhagic stroke

- **Haemorrhagic stroke.** This occurs when one or more of the vessels supplying the brain ruptures or bursts out, causing bleeding in the brain.

Still on the subject of strokes—I want us to look at what is referred to as **transient ischaemic attack (TIA)** or mini-stroke.

This involves a short-lived (usually less than 24 hours) disruption of blood supply to a part of the brain. Since the disruption is short-lived, so also is the disruption in the function of the affected part of the brain. This could be weakness of the limb, speech disruption, blurred vision etc. TIA does not lead to permanent brain damage. TIAs are important warning signs that could announce the occurrence of a full-blown stroke.

RISK FACTORS

Strokes and heart attacks share several common risk factors. These include:

- high blood pressure
- smoking
- obesity and
- inactivity.

SYMPTOMS

The symptoms of a stroke differ depending on the type of stroke and the part of the brain affected. The left half of the brain controls most of the activities of the right half of the body and the other way round. Thus a stroke affecting the left side of the brain could lead to loss of function on the right half of the body. The extent of loss of function depends on the extent of brain damage caused.

Symptoms usually set in suddenly, within seconds or minutes. Stroke and TIA symptoms may include:

- numbness, weakness or inability to move the face, arm or leg on one side of the body
- severe headache
- difficulty speaking
- sudden loss of sight in one eye or blurred vision
- confusion or difficulty understanding
- loss of balance or coordination
- seizures
- loss of consciousness

TREATMENT

The Creator fashioned our brain cells in such a way that once they have been damaged, they are irreparable. What can be done for a person who has suffered a stroke is to take measures to prevent another stroke or further strokes occurring in the future. Steps are therefore taken to treat the underlying cause of the stroke, for example high blood pressure.

In the acute phase of stroke, that is within the first 24-hours, treatment in a hospital, if available, is essential. I shall not go into the details of therapy here.

After the acute phase of therapy, the next stage is rehabilitation. It usually begins in the acute hospital, after about 48 hours of the occurrence.

The aim of rehabilitation is to help the patient relearn skills lost following the brain damage brought about by the stroke. These skills can include coordinating leg movements in order to walk or carrying out the steps involved in any complex activity. Rehabilitation also teaches survivors new ways of performing tasks to compensate for any disabilities brought about by the stroke.

Chapter 13

Asthma

∞

Asthma is a disease that affects the respiratory tract. In asthma, the airways of the affected person suddenly begins to narrow. The narrowing of the airways in turn leads to laboured breathing and wheezing. One can imagine a situation when someone attacks us, and with both hands attempts to suffocate us.

The number of individuals suffering from asthma has increased significantly over the last several years. Experts associate the new development with increased atmospheric pollution as well as changes in diet and lifestyle over the years.

ASTHMA RISK FACTORS AND TRIGGERS

- **Family History**: Asthma tends to occur in families. It is thought that about three-fifths of all asthma cases are hereditary. Thus if your mother or father has asthma, you are predisposed to having the condition.
- **Sex**: Childhood asthma occurs more frequently in boys than in girls. Around age 20, the ratio of asthma between men and women is the same. By age 40, more females than males have adult asthma.

- **Cigarette Smoke**: Actively smoking or inhaling the smoke exhaled from a smoker (passive smoking) can trigger asthma. (Passive smoking has even been identified as a risk factor for new cases of asthma in preschool-aged children who have not already exhibited asthma symptoms.)
- **Obesity**: Though the reason is unclear, evidence suggests that obesity may contribute to or even cause asthma. This is because the prevalence of asthma is increased in the obese or overweight individuals.
- **Exposure to Pollutants and Chemicals**: Exposure to environmental pollutants such as exhaust fumes as well as chemicals used in farming, hairdressing and manufacturing, etc., can serve as risk factors for the development of asthma as well as triggers of the condition in the affected individual.
- **Allergy.** Exposure to one or more of the substances listed below could trigger asthma in the individual allergic to them:

  1. House dust mites
  2. Mould spores
  3. Pollen
  4. Pets
  5. Food or food preservatives

- **Infection**: Viral or bacterial infection of the respiratory tract could serve as a trigger to an asthma attack.
- **Exercise:** Earlier in the book I mentioned the benefits of exercise to the body. For some individuals, exercise, especially vigorous exercise (in particular in cold air) could serve as a trigger for an asthma attack.

SYMPTOMS

- Shortness of breath that leads the affected person to gasp for air.

- Tightness of the chest, a situation that leads the affected person to feel as if there is a band tightening around the chest.
- Wheezing, which is a whistling sound heard on breathing, resulting from airflow obstruction secondary to the narrowing of the airwaves.
- Coughing, particularly at night and early morning.

TREATMENT

The goal of treatment is to restore the constricted airways back to its original form. Basically there are two types of drugs in use.

The first group act on the muscles of the constricted airways and cause them to relax, making it easier to breathe. These are also known as bronchodilators. The best known medication in this group is salbutamol.

The second group is made up of substances that act to reduce inflammation in the airways. This makes the airway less likely to react when exposed to asthma triggers. This group is made up mainly of steroids, for example beclomethasone.

Various combinations of the two types of substances are also available on the market.

In acute cases of asthma, the doctor may also dispense an injection with the goal of achieving swift relaxation of the respiratory muscles.

Where applicable, the doctor may also prescribe a short course of steroid tablets in an attempt to bring about a cure.

Chapter 14

Arthritis

∽

A rthritis is an inflammation of a joint. This can occur suddenly in a previously healthy joint. In this case medical science talks of acute arthritis. The condition may also persist after the initial manifestation. If this happens, the condition becomes chronic.

Chronic arthritis may cause the patient to experience episodes of worsening symptoms or flare-ups.

What is a joint?

Understanding the principles on which a joint is based will lead us to appreciate the amazing engineering capability of Almighty God.

We were not created to remain unmovable, like the mountains, but rather to move about and enjoy God's creation. To be able to do so, the Designer built joints, points of connection between two bones or elements of a skeleton into the skeleton system.

With a few exceptions, joints are designed to allow movement between the bones and to absorb shock from movements like walking or repetitive motion.

For the joints to move properly, Almighty God built a hard but slippery coating on the end of each bone, known as cartilage. Healthy cartilage

110

allows bones to glide over one another. It also absorbs energy from the shock of physical movement.

Next, He constructed a tough membrane sac, known as the joint capsule to enclose the bones and other joint parts.

Within the joint capsule is a thin membrane known as synovium. The synovium produces synovial fluid which serves the function of lubricating the joint to facilitate movement.

The entry of disease into God's perfect creation did not spare the joints. This brings me to the term *arthritis*, which, as I just mentioned, is an inflammation of a joint.

RIGHT KNEE   LEFT KNEE

Erosion of cartilage

Joint space narrowing

Bone spur

Eroding cartilage

Exposed bone

Eroding meniscus

Arthritis

Knee- joint changes in arthritis

There are two types of arthritis: osteoarthritis and rheumatoid arthritis.

OSTEOARTHRITIS

Also known as wear and tear arthritis, osteoarthritis is a disease which becomes more likely as persons get older.

In this condition the smooth cartilage that covers the end of bones begins to show signs of wear and tear. In the end, the fluid-filled space becomes smaller, causing the joint to be insufficiently lubricated. The wearing away of the joint cartilage may eventually expose the bone, leaving the surface of the now unprotected bone to rub directly against the opposing bone. This can lead to pain, in some cases severe or excruciating pain.

I try to explain osteoarthritis to my patients by comparing the human body to a brand new vehicle. Whoever has had the opportunity to drive a brand new automobile will have experienced the comfort of driving such a vehicle. In the first few months of its "life", it usually performs perfectly. In time, however, the brakes, the wipers, the clutch, etc., begin to show signs of wear and tear.

In the same vein, the human being, in his or her younger years, is usually fit and active. With the passing of time, however, his or her body begins to display signs of wear and tear, including the wear and tear of the joint surfaces.

Osteoarthritis most often occurs in the hands (at the ends of the fingers and thumbs), the spine (neck and lower back), and the knees, and hips.

RISK FACTORS IN OSTEOARTHRTIS

- **Age**: As was mentioned above, age is the main risk factor in the development of the condition.
- **Sex**: The condition is more common in women than in men.
- **Weight**: Being overweight increases the risk of osteoarthritis, in particular, osteoarthritis of the knee.
- **Previous injury:** an injury, surgery, earlier disease or repeated strain at a joint may lead to osteoarthritis later in life.

SYMPTOMS

Symptoms of osteoarthritis differ from individual to individual. Some people find the symptoms disabling whereas others may have few symptoms. Symptoms may include the following:

- **Stiffness** in a joint especially on getting out of bed or sitting for a long time.
- **Swelling** and inflammation in one or more joints.
- **Constant or recurring pain** in a joint.
- **Crunching feeling** or the sound of bone rubbing on bone.

DIAGNOSIS

Your doctor may use the following steps to confirm the condition:

- History taking
- Clinical examination
- Blood investigation
- X-ray
- MRI-scan.

TREATMENT

- **Medication**: There is no medication to treat the underlying disease process. Instead, the goal of medical treatment for osteoarthritis (OA) is to reduce pain and stiffness and make it easier to remain active. Analgesics (painkillers) and non-steroidal anti-inflammatory drugs (NSAIDs) are the most commonly prescribed osteoarthritis medicines.
- **Exercise**: Exercise, in particular, swimming, walking, and cycling, is known to have a favourable effect on alleviating the disease.

- **Weight control**: Weight reduction is important in the treatment of osteoarthritis. Weight loss can reduce the stress on weight-bearing joints, and in so doing limit injury and increase mobility.
- **Surgery**: In some patients surgery can help relieve pain and disability.
- **Use of prostheses**: In cases where joint degeneration has reached an advanced stage, surgeons may replace affected joints with artificial joints called prostheses. In general surgeons try to postpone the need for joint replacement as much as possible. Such joints usually last between 10 to 15 years; thereafter they need to be replaced.

RHEUMATOID ARTHRITIS (RA)

This is the second most common form of arthritis.

CAUSE

Earlier in the book, I explained the immune system placed at our disposal by Almighty God to defend us against infection and other diseases.

For reasons that cannot be explained the immune system sometimes turns against the same body it is there to defend. We may think of it as "friendly fire" as used in military jargon to describe the situation when an army fires accidentally on one of its own.

In the case of rheumatoid arthritis, the immune system attacks the tissues of the joints. This leads to inflammation of the joint. The inflammation causes swelling and redness in joints, and may make people feel sick, tired, and uncommonly feverish.

Persons suffering from rheumatic arthritis are subject to chronic joint pain with such acute recurrence that it can make their lives miserable. The joints eventually also become stiff, hampering smooth movement.

The most commonly affected joints are those at the ends of the fingers (closest to the nail), thumbs, neck, lower back, knees, and hips.

Compared with osteoarthritis, rheumatoid arthritis begins at a younger age than the former. It must be mentioned that apart from joints, rheumatoid arthritis can affect other parts of the body including the heart, lungs and digestive system.

RA can also occur in children. In this case, it is known as juvenile rheumatoid arthritis.

RISK FACTORS

- **Sex.** Women are more likely to develop rheumatoid arthritis than men.
- **Age.** As I just mentioned, rheumatoid arthritis can occur also in children. It is however most commonly observed in individuals between the ages of 30 and 60.
- **Family history.** As with many other medical conditions, one is at an increased risk of developing RA if other family members suffer from the condition.
- **Smoking.** Smoking has been identified as a risk factor for the development of RA.
- **Weight**: People who are obese or overweight are also at an increased risk of developing RA.

SYMPTOMS

- **Morning Stiffness:** A distinctive characteristic of rheumatoid arthritis is morning stiffness that lasts for at least an hour. In contrast the stiffness in osteoarthritis loosens up in about half an hour.
- **Swelling and Pain:** The joints swell up, turn warm and become tender. Indeed, swelling and pain in the joints must occur for at least 6 weeks before a diagnosis of rheumatoid arthritis is

considered. The joint symptoms occur symmetrically in pattern, for example both knees, both wrists, the corresponding fingers of both hands, but may be more severe on one side of the body (unlike osteoarthritis where only one joint may be affected).

- **Specific Joints Affected:** RA almost always develops in the wrists and knuckles (the knee and joints of the ball of the foot are often affected as well). Concerning the fingers, RA affects joints at the base of the fingers while sparing joints at the fingertips (osteoarthritis on its part affects the fingertips).
- **Nodules:** In some cases of RA, inflammation of small blood vessels can lead to the development of pea-size nodules, or lumps, under the skin, especially near the elbow area.
- **Fluid Build-up in joints:** RA may lead to the build-up of fluid in the joints, in particularly in the ankles.
- **Flu-like Symptoms:** In the early stages of the disease cold or flu-like symptoms, such as generalised bodily aches and pains, fatigue and fever may be felt by the affected person.
- **Anaemia:** The condition may lead to shortage of blood in the affected person.

Symptoms in Children

In children, juvenile rheumatoid arthritis is usually preceded by high fever and shaking chills along with pain and swelling in many joints. A pink skin rash may also be present.

TREATMENT

There is currently no cure for the condition. The aim of therapy in RA is to reduce inflammation in the joints, relieve pain, prevent or slow joint damage, reduce disability and provide support to help the affected person live as active a life as possible. This is achieved through the following:

MEDICATION

There are several groups of medication in use:

- Painkillers, eg Paracetamol.
- **Non-steroidal anti-inflammatory drugs (NSAIDs),** e.g. Diclofenac.
- **Corticosteroids** (Steroids are usually only used on a short-term basis, as long-term use can have serious side effects).
- **Disease-modifying anti-rheumatic drugs (DMARDs),** e.g. Methotrexate.
- **Biological Treatment**: Biological treatments are newer forms of treatment for rheumatoid arthritis. An example is the group of medication represented by the tumour necrosis factor-alpha (TNF-alpha) inhibitors such as infliximab.

NON-DRUG TREATMENT

Following are some of the popular non-drug therapies for arthritic pain relief. They may be used alone, or in combination.

- **Hot and cold treatments.** Usually applied directly to the pain site; heat may be more useful for chronic pain, and cold packs provide relief from acute pain.
- **Exercise.** Keeping your joints and muscles moving helps in general fitness and can lead to decrease in pain.
- **Massage.** Massage can lead to relaxation of muscles and provide some arthritic pain relief.
- **Electrical stimulation.** Also known as transcutaneous electrical nerve stimulation (TENS), the therapy is delivered through a small device that sends a painless electrical current to large nerve fibres, generating heat that relieves stiffness and pain. The current also stimulates the release of endorphins, the body's natural painkillers.

LIFESTYLE CHANGES

The following lifestyle changes may favourably influence the course of the disease:

- A good and healthy diet.
- Losing weight in case of obesity.
- Smoking cessation.

SURGERY

Surgical treatment is employed in rheumatoid arthritis to relieve severe pain and improve the function of severely deformed joints that do not respond to medication and physical therapy. In some cases surgery may involve total joint replacement (arthroplasty).

Chapter 15

Diabetes

O ne day a middle-aged woman consulted me in my practice and began:

"Doc, I think there is something wrong with me."

"What then?"

"I have been feeling increasingly thirsty. Indeed, I am forced to drink almost all the time. That is not the end of the matter—I must frequently pass urine as well. It appears as if I have to drink water only to pass it out as urine!"

At this point in her narration the alarm bells, as it were, began to ring in my head. I was almost certain what was wrong with her; I wouldn't tell her immediately, however.

"There is certainly something wrong with you. We shall have to find out. You seem to have lost some weight as well."

"That is certainly the case. I have lost a few kilograms over the last several days. No wonder, for I have lost my appetite. I also feel tired all the time. Please Doc, help me, for matters certainly cannot continue like this!"

By now I knew exactly what her symptoms pointed to, namely, diabetes—what in several languages including my native Twi language is referred to as "sugar disease".

Knowing the type of person she was, I did not want to reveal my suspicions to her without first substantiating them with the relevant tests.

"We will have to conduct a few tests to find out what is wrong with you—first, you will need to provide us with a urine sample; next, we shall examine your blood."

"That's fine, Doc; I hope we are able to get to the bottom of the matter soon."

"We will do our best," I assured her.

As I expected, the tests confirmed my suspicion. Indeed, her symptoms were very typical of the onset of diabetes.

What, then, is Diabetes?

I shall explain it from the Christian perspective.

Almighty God placed us on the planet earth for a purpose. To go about our activities, we would need energy. He created plants and animals to provide us with food. Through the process of digestion, the foodstuffs we eat are broken down into three basic components: glucose, amino acid, and fatty acid. These are eventually absorbed into our bloodstream.

We might consider glucose as a kind of fuel—petrol, diesel, or kerosene—that needs to be burned to power our body systems. For glucose to be effective, it must move into the cells to power the various reactions going on there.

To make this possible, Almighty God placed at our disposal the pancreas. Weighing approximately eighty grams, it is located behind the stomach. The pancreas serves two main functions. In the first place, it produces enzymes that help in the digestion of foodstuffs once they pass from the stomach into the small intestine.

Most importantly, however, it produces two substances—insulin and glucagon, that help to regulate the level of glucose in the blood. Without doubt, insulin, which helps to transport glucose from the bloodstream to the cells, is the more important of the two.

After we have eaten to our fill and digestion and absorption has led to an elevation of the level of glucose in our bloodstream, the pancreas receives an order from the brain to release insulin into our bloodstream. The insulin so released picks up the glucose circulating in the bloodstream for onward transport to the cells, like the letter carrier picking up our letters from the post office and depositing them in our letterboxes.

By means of one stone, insulin, the pancreas seeks to kill two birds. Firstly, it reduces the concentration of sugar levels in the blood and by so doing averts the harm that such high concentrations could have on the body in the end. Secondly, insulin ensures that the glucose reaches the parts of the body that need it, mainly, inside the cells.

In diabetes, or "sugar disease", the pancreas may either completely cease to produce insulin or may not produce insulin in a sufficient quantity. It may well be the case that the body cells of the affected person cannot react properly to insulin produced by the pancreas.

In a person suffering from **Type1 Diabetes** the cells in the pancreas responsible for insulin production are destroyed. It is thought by medical science that the destruction of the pancreas cells is due to an autoimmune disease (remember what I said earlier when I explained the immune system). It is thought that a virus infection or an environmental factor serves as a trigger to spark the autoimmune reaction.

In the case of **Type 2 Diabetes**, either the pancreas cannot produce enough insulin or the body cells of the affected person cannot react properly to insulin.

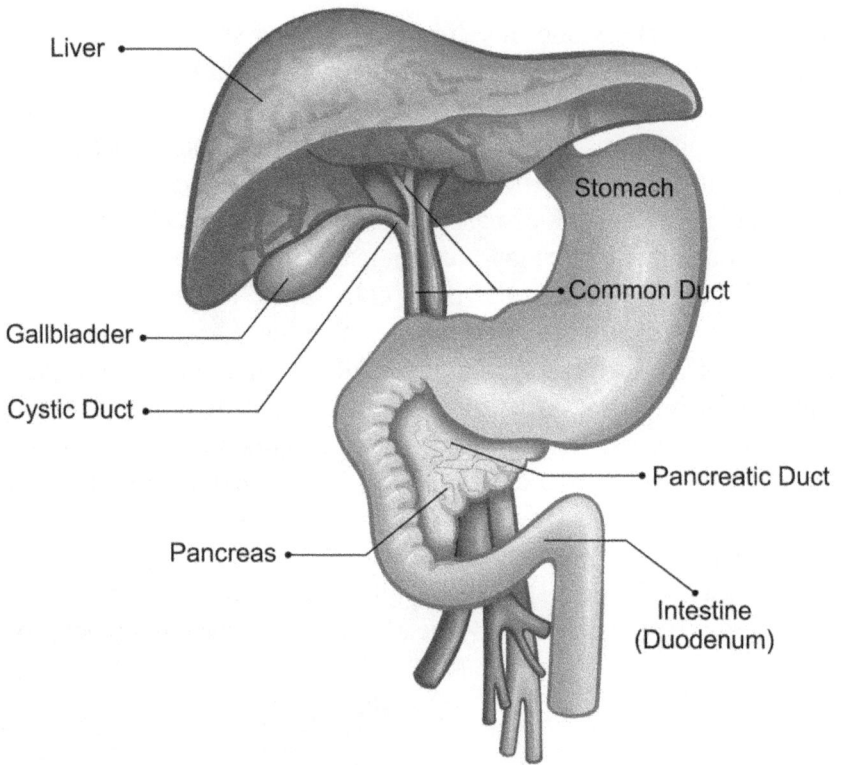

Position of the pancreas in the body

RISK FACTORS FOR TYPE 2 DIABETES

- **Obesity**: Obesity or being overweight is a major risk factor for the development of Diabetes Type 2. Previously, the condition was generally associated with adults. As the number of overweight children increases in many societies, so also, unfortunately, does the number of children who increasingly are being diagnosed with the condition.
- **Lack of exercise**: With the advent of automobiles, the remote control, the computer, computer games, etc., we have increasingly

become inactive. Inactivity coupled with the availability of abundant food in our refrigerators may lead us to overfeeding which in turn could lead to overweight which in turn could lead to the development of Type 2 Diabetes.

- **Unhealthy eating habits**: Earlier I touched on the concept of a balanced diet. Bad or unhealthy eating habits—eating too much fat, too much carbohydrate (starchy food), and not enough fibre increases the risk of developing Type 2 diabetes.
- **Family history:** As in the case of high blood pressure, diabetes seems to occur in families. It does not follow automatically that because your father or mother has the condition you are also going to get it. You only need to remember that you are more susceptible to getting it in order to adopt a healthier lifestyle.
- **Gestational Diabetes:** Some women develop diabetes during pregnancy. This is also known as *gestational diabetes*. In the majority of cases, the condition returns to normal after birth. Studies have shown that these women stand the risk of developing Type 2 diabetes later in life. Such women are thus advised to avoid exposing themselves to the risks just outlined.
- **High Blood Pressure**: As I mentioned in the chapter on high blood pressure, the two conditions seem to go together. If you have been diagnosed with high blood pressure, your risk of developing Type 2 diabetes is higher than that of the general population.

SYMPTOM

As we saw earlier, my patient presented us with some of the typical symptoms of the disease. These include:

- Feeling thirsty all the time.
- Having to pass urine all the time.
- Weight loss.
- Feeling tired and exhausted.
- Loss of appetite.

TREATMENT

Type 1:
As we learnt above, in the person with Type 1 diabetes, the body cannot produce insulin at all. Treatment is by way of insulin. Insulin, when taken in tablet form, is destroyed by acids in the stomach. Consequently, the main route of application is by means of injection. Attempts are being made to produce insulin that can be inhaled so as to spare victims the need to inject insulin.

Type 2 Diabetes:
As we saw earlier, in patients with Type 2 diabetes, the pancreas is either not producing sufficient insulin to meet the demands of the body, or the body cells cannot react properly to insulin (medical science speaks in this case also of insulin-resistance).

Treatment in this case is by means of tablets that help to activate the remaining pancreatic cells to increase insulin production. Some of these patients may have to inject insulin in addition to taking the tablets.

We learnt about the risk factors in developing the disease. In some instances blood sugar levels can be restored to normal levels without even the need for medication. Instead, the patient takes steps to reduce the risk factors that lead to the condition—reducing weight, following the proper diet and undertaking regular exercise.

LONG TERM EFFECT OF DIABETES

Diabetes that isn't well controlled can lead to long-term problems for the patient. The elevated blood glucose associated with the condition can lead to the damage of blood vessels which in turn can lead to: heart and kidney disease, stroke, impotence and nerve damage.

Chapter 16

Epilepsy

⊂⊃

At the time I was growing up in my little village, one of our fellow residents suffered from epilepsy. The great majority of the population were either completely illiterate or at best semi-educated. Hardly anyone of us had any idea as to the underlying cause of the disease. Consequently we fell victim to the then prevailing belief that the disease could be passed on to anyone who happened to come too close to the afflicted person at the time he or she was experiencing a fit. Thus, whenever the victim of the disease suffered a fit, whoever happened to be near him, made for the hills instead of going to his or her aid.

CAUSES

The Creator God has placed billions of nerve cells in our brains. The nerve cells transmit impulses from one to the other. They do so by way of chemicals known as neurotransmitters. There are two types of neurotransmitters; one type leads to an increase in impulse transmission, whereas the other inhibits the process. In normal life the activities of the two transmitters are co-ordinated in such a manner as to lead to stability in brain activity. A disturbance in the delicate balance could lead to epileptic fits.

RISK FACTORS

Below are some of the factors that can bring about a disturbance in the delicate balance in neurotransmitter activity in the brain alluded to above.

- **Genetic abnormality:** Medical science has observed that some types of epilepsy tend to run in families. This has led to the suspicion of genetic abnormality as one possible cause of the disease.
- **Head injury:** Head injuries sustained in accidents may lead to seizures or epileptic fits. This is particularly so when the injuries involved happen to be severe.
- **Prenatal injuries:** When we are developing in our mother's womb, our brain cells are very susceptible to adverse changes in the womb environment brought about either by maternal illness or behaviour. For example, some types of infection contracted by an expectant mother, or habits such as smoking, alcohol consumption as well as the abuse of certain drugs, if continued through the pregnancy, can adversely affect the unborn child and lead eventually to epilepsy in later years.
- **Environmental factors:** Exposure to lead, carbon monoxide, and certain chemicals, should it persist for a considerable period, could lead to the development of epilepsy.
- **Alcohol:** Long-standing alcohol abuse can increase a person's risk of developing epilepsy.
- **Disease:** Epilepsy can be a secondary manifestation of a primary condition such as brain tumour, meningitis, HIV, etc.
- **Other factors:** sleep deprivation and stress could lead to epileptic fits in an individual.

TREATMENT

Medication: There are several groups of medication in use for the treatment of epilepsy. Treatment depends on several factors including the age of the affected person, how often the seizures occur, how severe they are as well as the overall health of the affected person. Readers are advised to contact their own doctors in regard to the treatment options available.

Surgery: In some instances surgery, the details of which I shall spare the reader, is employed in the treatment of epilepsy.

Chapter 17

Sexually Transmitted Diseases

∞

Earlier on in the book, I outlined examples of sexually transmitted diseases. In this chapter, I will look at each condition in some detail.

CHLAMYDIA

Chlamydia is caused by the bacterium, Chlamydia trachomatis. The disease can affect women and men as well as children during their passage through the birth canal. Symptoms usually appear approximately 7 to 21 days after infection and differ for men, women and children.

In men Chlamydia can cause inflammation of the urethra (the passage through which urine passes to the outside of the body). This in turn can result in a stinging feeling when passing water. The disease can also lead to a discharge from the male genital organ and possible itchiness as well as pain. Finally it could also lead to pain in the testicles.

As in men, the disease can also lead to a stinging feeling in women when passing water as well as being accompanied by unusual genital discharge.

The disease can lead the affected female to experience pain during intercourse as well as experience bleeding between periods.

Infection in an expectant mother could lead to premature birth.

Infants can contract the disease during birth. An infection could lead to the following symptoms: conjunctivitis (inflammation of the eye), breathing problems, chest infection (pneumonia).

DIAGNOSIS

Diagnosis is done by performing a swab test of the infected area and examining it in the laboratory for evidence of infection.

TREATMENT

This is by means of suitable antibiotics, eg Doxycycline and Zithromax. It is recommended that the spouse of the affected person is also treated.

GONORRHOEA

The condition is caused by bacteria called Neisseria gonorrhoeae. It can affect both sexes. In women, the cervix or the neck of the womb is the most common site of infection. The disease can also spread to the uterus (womb) and fallopian tubes. This can lead to the blockage of the fallopian tubes which in turn can lead to infertility!

In women the early symptoms of gonorrhoea are often mild, and many women who are infected have no visible symptoms of the disease.

In the female symptoms include: a painful, burning sensation when urinating, a yellowish or bloody discharge from the genital organ, inter-menstrual bleeding and abdominal pain.

Symptoms in the male are clearer than in the female. They include a burning sensation when passing urine and a yellowish-white discharge from the male genital organ.

Gonorrhoea can be passed from an affected expectant mother to her new-born infant during delivery.

DIAGNOSIS

Diagnosis is made through detection of bacteria in samples taken from the urethra or cervix.

TREATMENT

The condition is treated with antibiotics such as penicillin, cefixime and ciprofloxacin. Treatment should be extended to the spouse of the affected person. As with Chlamydia, further testing is recommended once treatment has ended to check whether the infection has cleared

HERPES GENITALIS

This is caused by the herpes simplex virus (HSV). It is a highly contagious condition. It is transmitted primarily through physical and sexual contact. During birth, an infected mother can pass the condition on to the new-born during his/her passage through the birth canal. This could lead among others to the development of herpetic meningitis.

SYMPTOMS

The outbreak may be accompanied by other symptoms such as:

- Swelling and tenderness of the lymph nodes in the groin area.
- In women, vaginal discharge and painful urination.
- In men, a possibility of painful urination if the lesion is near the opening of the urethra.
- Fever.

TREATMENT

There is no cure for the herpes simplex virus; once infected, patients will remain a carrier for the rest of their lives. Timely treatment (within five days of symptoms starting) with antiviral medication will reduce the severity and duration of symptoms. A five-day course of treatment is usual, but may be extended by a few days if blisters are still forming. Examples of this group of medication are aciclovir, famciclovir and valaciclovir.

HIV/AIDS

HIV has become a household name. HIV invades and destroys the immune system, which as I have mentioned in several places in this book, was put in place in our body by Almighty God to, among other things, protect the body from infection. The result of this is that the affected person becomes prone to many different types of diseases.

We might well imagine what would happen to a country should it be invaded by outside forces, just at the very point in time when its entire military force is incapacitated by disease.

RISK FACTORS

The virus is found in bodily fluids such as blood, sperm and vaginal secretions, and can pass through little scratches that may be present or occur during sexual intercourse. Consequently intravenous drug users and people with many different partners are particularly at risk of contracting the disease.

SYMPTOMS

Although they vary considerably, the symptoms include:

- fever
- diarrhoea
- night sweats
- weight loss
- swollen glands
- the feeling of being generally unwell.

DIAGNOSIS

The diagnosis is made when the HIV antibody is found in the blood. The test is not usually positive until 6 to 12 weeks after infection.

TREATMENT

That HIV has until now no effective cure is a well-known fact, and may be superfluous to mention here. Therapy currently is aimed at the improvement of the quality of life and its prolongation. Several medications aimed at achieving this are currently on the market. It is beyond the scope of this book to look at the various types of medication in detail.

GENITAL WARTS

Also known as condylomata acuminate, it is a very contagious condition caused by the human papilloma virus (HPV). As we shall see later when we come to treat cancer, some strains of this virus can lead to changes in the cervix which in turn can lead to the development of cervical cancer. Up to nine months can pass from the time of infection to the actual development of warts. About a third of cases of genital warts may resolve without treatment after six months. Rarely, they can develop into cauliflower-like growths.

SYMPTOMS

These include the following:

- Red, pink or grey-coloured cauliflower-shaped lesions in the genital and anal area that look raised or flat. The abnormal growths may develop into large clusters and expand into huge masses very rapidly.
- Tiny papules on the shaft of the penis.
- Discomfort and itching in the affected areas.

- Mild cases of warts are usually painless. In severe cases, they may cause severe pain.

DIAGNOSIS

A diagnosis is made when a characteristic lesion is visible. By swabbing the skin with 5 per cent acetic acid, 'invisible' warts will emerge as white-coloured patches.

TREATMENT

Treatment of genital warts depends on their size and location.

- Chemicals such as imiquimod and podophyllotoxin may be used to remove visible warts.
- Cryotherapy : This involves the freezing of genital warts, using liquid nitrogen.
- Where available, laser therapy can be used.
- Surgery can be used to remove the genital wart, in particular those that have assumed large sizes.

SYPHILIS

The disease is caused by bacteria called Treponema pallidum. The route of transmission of syphilis is almost always through sexual contact though it can also be transmitted from mother to child in the womb or during birth.

It can be potentially life-threatening because after infection, the bacteria is transported through the bloodstream to various parts of the body. In the end it could adversely affect vital organs such as the heart, brain, nervous system and spine.

DIAGNOSIS

This is made through the detection of the micro-organism or the detection of antibodies in the blood.

SYMPTOMS AND STAGES OF DISEASE

There are three stages of the disease:

- Stage 1: This occurs up to the first twelve weeks of the infection. During this period one or more red lesions could be observed in the genital area. The lesions usually disappear after a week.
- Stage 2: Symptoms could be observed up to about six months after the time of infection. These may include the following: a red rash on the chest, back, arms, legs, hands and soles of the feet; high fever; muscular fatigue as well as a general feeling of discomfort.
- Stage 3: If the disease is not identified and treated, it will disappear for a while only to return later, sometimes up to twenty years later. At this more advanced stage of the diseases, the symptoms could include heart failure, paralysis, insanity which in turn could lead to the death of the patient. (If we sit down to consider the fact that the disease we contracted several years ago through sexual contact could cause us serious problems twenty years later we would indeed make every effort to keep the temple of God that we indeed are holy.)

TREATMENT

Syphilis: is treated with penicillin, administered by injection. Other antibiotics can be used for patients allergic to penicillin. Left untreated, it could damage the heart, the brain, eyes and bones. In some cases these effects could lead to death.

PART 4

WOMEN'S HEALTH

Chapter 18

Menstrual Disorders

∽

I n this chapter I will deal with menstrual problems and problems related to menopause. Before I do that, I shall take some time to explain the menstrual cycle from the Christian perspective.

The question to consider at the outset is this: why is there a need for a menstrual cycle in the first place?

Almighty God in His wisdom, decided to cooperate with humankind in the propagation of the human race. In the end He decided on the principle of division of labour, assigning the male and the female different functions of sexual reproduction.

Among other things, He assigned the female the role of carrying the new individual resulting from the union of the egg and the sperm and providing the child the opportunity to develop and grow in her womb until such time that the baby is capable of surviving under the prevailing conditions on earth.

To facilitate the performance of the role assigned to her, Almighty God instituted the female menstrual cycle.

In our present discussion, we will assume an average duration of twenty-eight days, although it may deviate a few days from individual to individual.

The cycle in effect is the female body's way of preparing itself to accommodate the would-be product of the union referred to above. The expected union not having materialised, the womb decides, albeit with a heavy heart, to discard the material put in place to receive the newcomer.

Depending on the individual involved, the menstrual bleeding may last anywhere between three and seven days (or more). When the bleeding is over, the brain sends instructions to a structure located at its base, the pituitary gland, to begin releasing into the bloodstream a hormone it had all along been producing and storing in its body. This hormone on its part carries the name follicle-stimulating hormone, or FSH. FSH in turn instructs one of the two ovaries of the womb to order one of the several follicles it is harbouring to grow into maturity. The follicles are tiny liquid-filled sacs, each containing an egg. At birth, each girl already has several follicles. They remain dormant until she reaches maturity.

Usually during each menstrual cycle, only one follicle grows into maturity. In rare instances, however, two or more may do so simultaneously and release their eggs into the womb.

Mechanism of ovulation in the menstrual cycle

There are two ovaries on each side of the womb. For the sake of fairness, the follicles release at alternating months from each ovary.

Prior to the release of the matured egg into the womb, the maturing follicle releases a considerable amount of a hormone known as oestrogen into the bloodstream. Under the influence of oestrogen, the lining of the womb grows increasingly thicker.

Just about the middle of the 28-day cycle, that is, round about the fourteenth day, the matured egg drops into the womb. We call this event ovulation.

The important role the follicle plays does not end with ovulation. Now re-christened corpus luteum, it begins to release, in addition to oestrogen, another hormone, progesterone, into the bloodstream. Together, both hormones support and maintain the thickened walls of the uterus in anticipation of the possible implantation of the fertilised egg within it.

In the absence of fertilisation, the corpus luteum degenerates in about fourteen days. With decreasing levels of oestrogen and progesterone in the bloodstream brought about by the degeneration of the corpus luteum, a new menstrual cycle soon sets in.

I believe that in the world prior to the fall of humanity, the menstrual cycle went on without any discomfort, pain or distress to the woman.

And God saw everything that he had made, and, behold, it was very good. And the evening and the morning were the sixth day. Genesis 1:31

At the moment however Mankind is wandering in the Sinai desert far removed from the Land of Promise. So headaches, suffering and thorns continue to afflict us.

Unto the woman he said, I will greatly multiply thy sorrow and thy conception; in sorrow thou shalt bring forth children; and thy desire shall be to thy husband, and he shall rule over thee. Genesis 3:16

This leads to some of the common problems and disturbances that could affect the menstrual cycle.

AMENORRHEA

The age of onset of menstruation in a girl varies from individual to individual, depending on several factors. Some girls start menstruation as early as 8 years whereas others have to wait until they are around 16 years of age.

It is generally agreed that by the age of 16 every girl would have experienced her first menstruation.

If this does not happen, the resulting condition is referred to by medical science as primary amenorrhea.

There are instances when a girl /woman who has all along not had any problem with her period, all of a sudden stops to menstruate. If this condition persists for six consecutive months, the doctors refer to the condition as secondary amenorrhoea. (One has to keep in mind that it may well be due to a pregnancy, of course.)

DYSMENORRHEA

A certain degree of pain or discomfort accompanies even the normal menstrual cycle. Medical science speaks of dysmenorrhea or menstrual pain when the discomfort and pain is bad enough to interfere with the normal daily life of the individual concerned.

The pain typically occurs in the lower abdomen and/or pelvis and can radiate to the back and along the thighs, lasting somewhere between 8 and 72 hours. It may be a constant dull ache or occur as cramps before or during menstruation or both. Headaches, diarrhoea, nausea and vomiting may accompany it.

Severe menstrual pain can be a sign of an underlying disease such as endometriosis and fibroids.

In endometrioses, the cells that line the cavity of the womb and that are shed during each menstrual cycle, are also found in places outside of the womb. During each menstrual period, the tissue outside of the womb, like that inside the womb, responds to the hormones that regulate the menstrual cycle. This leads to a breakdown and bleeding of the tissue in the same way as those lining the walls of the womb. This can lead to inflammation and pain.

MENORRHAGIA

This refers to prolonged or excessive menstrual bleeding that occurs at regular intervals. In most cases no cause can be found. However, there may be an underlying cause such as endometriosis, fibroids or even womb cancer.

INTERMENSTRUAL BLEEDING OR SPOTTING

This refers to bleeding of variable amounts that occur between regular menstrual periods. These may have several causes including hormonal imbalance, infection, fibroids, etc.

POLYMENORRHEA

In this case bleeding occurs in regular intervals of less than 21 days.

OLIGOMENORRHOEA

This is irregular or infrequent periods. Menstruation can occur anywhere between every six weeks and six months.

PREMENSTRUAL SYNDROM (PMS)

Premenstrual Syndrom, PMS for short, is a condition that occurs about ten to fourteen days before the onset of menstruation. It involves physical and emotional symptoms that may include bloating, pressure on the pelvis, headaches or migraines, difficulty concentrating, irritability, mood swings and increased craving for food.

The degree to which PMS occurs is different from woman to woman— some women may experience none, some, or many PMS symptoms. Also for each individual woman, the symptoms may be worse in some months than others.

For the Christian woman, I do identify a call to prayer here, for the evil one can manipulate the condition for his own good, a situation that could lead among other things to an emotional state in which the woman can easily become angry with those who come into contact with her.

Chapter 19

Fibroids

A s I stated earlier, Almighty God in His own wisdom decided to co-operate with Humankind in the multiplication of our race.

The woman was given the responsibility to keep and nurture the developing baby in the womb until he or she was in a position to live an independent life. To make that possible, Almighty God placed the womb, which can be described as a muscular sack, at the disposal of the woman to serve as home for the developing baby.

The womb of a woman, known as the uterus, when not pregnant, measures about 8 cm in length, 5 cm in width and about 2.5 cm in thickness. The extent of expansion that this small mass of muscle undergoes in order to harbour the unborn child is simply incredible!

The womb was not spared the effect of the Divine Curse pronounced on our original parents in the Garden of Eden. This brings me to the matter of fibroids.

Also known as myomas, fibroids are benign (not cancerous) tumours found in the muscular wall of the uterus.

They are quite common, occurring in about a third of all women. Many of the affected women live with it without knowing it, for indeed in many cases fibroids are not accompanied by any symptoms. That, unfortunately, is not the case for all women, for fibroids do cause problems for many.

CAUSES

Medical science has not been able to explain exactly why some women develop fibroids and others do not. There is general consensus among the experts however as to the role of the hormone oestrogen.

Oestrogen plays an important role in the function of the female body. The level of oestrogen falls after the menopause. It has been observed that the size of fibroids in women decreases after the menopause. This has led to the conclusion that oestrogen, even if it does not cause it, at least facilitates the growth of fibroids.

Fibroids vary in their location, shape and size. Also, whereas some women develop a single fibroid which may assume large sizes, others develop many small fibroids.

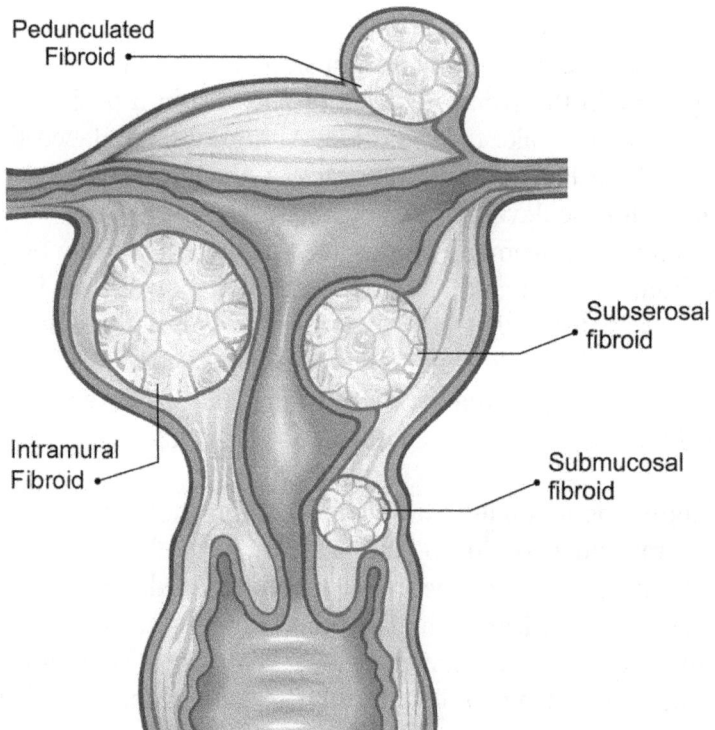

Types of Fibroids

TYPES

Based on their location relative to the womb, fibroids are divided into four main types:

- **Submucous fibroids**. These grow in the hollow space within the womb. By virtue of their location this types of fibroid can adversely affect a pregnancy. This is especially the case should the pregnancy implant on it. In such a situation the fetus is in danger of not receiving an adequate blood supply which in turn could lead to a miscarriage. Ultimately, submucous fibroids could result in infertility of the affected woman.
- **Intramural fibroids**: Theses are fibroids located within the muscle of the uterine wall.
- **Extramual**: This type of fibroid grows on the outside wall of the womb.
- **Pedunculated fibroids:** These kinds of fibroids develop on a 'stalk' or stem-like structure attached to the inside or the outside of the uterus. These fibroids can become twisted, leading to severe pain and heavy bleeding.

SYMPTOMS

What are the signs that point to fibroids? As I mentioned earlier, in several women they produce no symptoms at all. Usually they begin to cause problems when they assume large sizes. (That is not to say that small fibroids do not cause problems.)

Menstrual Disturbances

They can be in the form of:

- Increased menstrual bleeding which in turn can lead to anaemia.
- Prolonged menstrual bleeding.
- Increased menstrual frequency.
- Inter-menstrual bleeding (bleeding between the normal menstrual period).

Abdominal Pain

Fibroids, particularly large ones, may lead to bloating and/ or abdominal discomfort.

Low Back Pain

Fibroids that have assumed large sizes can lead to (lower) back pain.

Urinary Problems

The womb lies not far from the urinary bladder. Fibroids, in particular large fibroids, may result in the compression of the urinary bladder which in turn can lead the woman to urinate frequently.

Constipation

Fibroids can also occur on the rectum (the end of the large intestine) and lead to constipation.

Other related problems

Huge fibroids may create the impression of the affected person being pregnant. In some societies it could lead to all sorts of rumours among neighbours, particularly if it is not treated early. One can imagine the psychological impact that it could have on the affected woman.

Problems with childbirth

As I mentioned above, fibroids, especially those found within the womb, can cause problems in the pregnancy, especially so when the pregnancy implants on it.

This can lead to inadequate blood supply to the fetus which in turn can lead to miscarriage. In the end this type of fibroid can lead to infertility.

Even if it does not lead to infertility, they can lead to complications during the pregnancy. These can be in the form of threatened miscarriage, miscarriage, premature delivery, etc.

Fibroids, if they are located in the birth canal, can, make normal delivery impossible.

DIAGNOSIS

This is mainly by means of a clinical examination (pelvic examination) followed by an ultrasound scan (if available).

TREATMENT

Most fibroids do not require treatment. Treatment is usually needed if the fibroids are causing some of the symptoms listed above, pain or bleeding, or if the fibroids are large or rapidly growing.

Medication

Some types of medication act on the fibroids with the aim of reducing their size and preventing them from growing any further. Other types of medication are used to treat the bleeding associated with the condition.

Surgery

Surgery is considered where medication does not lead to the expected results.

The choice of surgery depends on the type and size of the fibroid and include:

- Myomectomy: This involves the removal of the fibroid and the preservation of the womb. This path is usually pursued where the fibroids involved are small and also where the woman desires to have children. (The fibroids may return at a later date, however.)
- Hysterectomy: This involves the complete removal of the uterus.

Chapter 20

Female Infertility

⌒◯⌒

And God blessed them, and God said unto them, Be fruitful, and multiply, and replenish the earth, and subdue it: and have dominion over the fish of the sea, and over the fowl of the air, and over every living thing that moveth upon the earth. Genesis 1:28
   Lo, children are an heritage of the LORD: and the fruit of the womb is his reward. Psalm 127:3

If a couple should fail to conceive during a year of unprotected intercourse, medical science refers to the couple as being infertile. Infertility can be caused by a problem with the man or the woman, or both.

Female reproductive problems account for 40 per cent of all cases of infertility, while 40 per cent are assigned to the male. In the remaining 20 per cent, medical science is at a loss as to the cause.

Yet, in several societies, the female is usually the first person assigned blame when couples find it difficult to conceive.

In my native Ghana, the pressure on the female can, in such a situation, be enormous. We have a family set up that can be regarded as a community. Children are not looked upon as belonging to the couple involved but to the community, the extended family as a whole. When a marriage after a while fails to produce children, the extended family members of both individuals have a tendency, sooner rather than later, to point accusing fingers at the woman.

In this chapter I will consider some of the factors that may lead to female infertility. Male infertility will be treated in the following chapter.

CAUSES OF FEMALE INFERTILITY

OVULATION PROBLEMS

It takes two to tango! The sperm of the male may be active, agile and willing to tango with the egg of the female, but if the eggs are absent in the womb at the time Mr Sperm gets there no tango can take place.

Eggs are released by the female in the process of ovulation. What factors can lead to problems of ovulation?

One of the culprits identified is the so-called Polycystic Ovary Syndrome (PCOS). This condition affects about 5% to 10% of women of reproductive age. Some of the features present in a female displaying signs of the syndrome are obesity (overweight), female masculinisation (when women display features that make them appear to look like men), acne, irregular periods, inability to ovulate. How far the above symptoms develop in an individual is different from woman to woman.

TUBAL PROBLEMS

After ovulation, Princess Egg needs to travel through the fallopian tube to meet Prince Sperm to join together in holy matrimony. In some instances, several factors working either alone or together prevent that from happening.

Following are some of the factors that may cause problems to the egg in its journey through the fallopian tube:

- Endometrioses
- Pelvic adhesions
- Pelvic Inflammatory Disease
- Blocked Fallopian tube

UTERINE PROBLEMS

After Mr Sperm and Miss Egg have sealed their marriage bond, they need a home to settle in and develop their relations. The uterus comes into play here. Several conditions in the uterus can either prevent this from happening; if in their attempt to settle in the womb their peace is disturbed by unruly elements, the new residents may decide, prematurely, to vacate their new residence (leading to miscarriage).

One of the conditions in the uterus that could lead to such a situation is the presence of fibroids. Fibroids, in particular those within the womb, as we noted earlier, can lead among other things to the improper implantation of the fetus on the wall of the womb and lead to miscarriage, not only of one pregnancy but several others.

AGE-RELATED FACTORS

And he said, I will certainly return unto thee according to the time of life; and, lo, Sarah thy wife shall have a son. And Sarah heard it in the tent door, which was behind him. Now Abraham and Sarah were old and well stricken in age; and it ceased to be with Sarah after the manner of women. Therefore Sarah laughed within herself, saying, After I am waxed old shall I have pleasure, my Lord being old also? And the LORD said unto Abraham, Wherefore did Sarah laugh, saying, Shall I of a surety bear a child, which am old? Is anything too hard for the LORD? At the time appointed I will return unto thee, according to the time of life, and Sarah shall have a son. Genesis 18: 10-14

I do believe that with God all things are possible. He can indeed intervene, in supernatural ways, to change the course of events, just as in the above passage

In normal life circumstances, we know that a time comes in the life the female when she is no longer in a position to conceive. Even several years before the menopause, it usually becomes increasingly difficult for a woman to conceive.

DIAGNOSIS

A doctor suspecting female infertility would do the following to confirm his/her suspicion (I shall leave out the details):

- History, including menstrual and pregnancy history
- Clinical examination
- Blood investigation
- Ovulation tests
- Laparoscopy (to determine endometrioses and adhesion)

TREATMENT

Lo, children are an heritage of the LORD: and the fruit of the womb is his reward. Psalm 127:3

Much as we are called upon to pray about everything, it is even more imperative to do so when it comes to the issue of difficulty in conceiving. In 1 Samuel 1:1-2:11 we learn of how Hannah asked the Lord for a child and how the Lord heard her prayer, leading to the birth of Samuel.

As far as medical science is concerned, the following are some of the treatment options:

- **Induction of Ovulation**. If the inability to ovulate is the cause of infertility, the doctor will prescribe medication with the goal of overcoming the problem.
- **Intrauterine Insemination**: This is a fertility procedure whereby sperm are washed, concentrated and injected directly into a woman's uterus. In natural intercourse, only a portion of the sperm are able to travel up the woman's genital tract

to the fallopian tube to bring about fertilisation. Intrauterine insemination increases the number of sperm in the fallopian tube; that in turn increases the chance of fertilisation taking place.

- **IVF**: This is a term which in the meantime has become generally known. You may speak to your doctor about the details.

Chapter 21

Pregnancy-related issues

∽

NORMAL COURSE OF A PREGNANCY

Someone has said that at the time of our birth we are already nine months old. This is indeed true, for from the moment of conception, the complex genetic blueprint for every detail of human development—sex, hair and eye colour, height, and skin tone—are already mapped out.

By approximately the fifth week of the union, the individual's heart has begun to beat. By the end of the fourth week, the spinal cord, muscles, and nerves have become apparent; so also the arms, legs, eyes, and ears.

During the last six months of pregnancy organ systems continue to refine themselves.

At the end of nine months the incredible events are complete and a child is about to be born. The normal position for the baby as it prepares for birth is head down and facing the mother's back.

SIGNS AND SYMPTOMS OF A NORMAL PREGNANCY

Having spoken of the normal course of pregnancy by way of introduction, I shall now move on to outline some of the common signs and symptoms of a normal pregnancy.

It should be noted that symptoms may vary from woman to woman; also, some of the symptoms are similar to the discomforts that a woman may experience prior to a normal menstruation.

Missed Period: This is the most obvious early pregnancy symptom. This could be caused by other medical conditions, but if it is followed soon by some of the symptoms outlined below, it is likely due to a pregnancy.

Breast Tenderness: A tender, swollen and a slightly sore breast. Some women may also notice their nipples darken in colour.

Nausea and Vomiting: Nausea and vomiting, especially in the morning, may be experienced very early in the pregnancy, as early as a week into the pregnancy.

Fatigue, Dizziness and Fainting: For some women one of the early signs of pregnancy is the feeling of being tired for the most part of the day. While this may force them to go to bed early, they may also find it difficult to wake up in the morning.

In addition to feeling tired all the time, some women may also often feel dizzy and feel like passing out.

Frequent Urination: Pregnancy results in an increase in body fluids that has to be processed by the kidneys. The expansion of the uterus, on its part, exerts constant pressure on the urinary bladder. Both factors together lead to frequent urination of the pregnant woman.

Heartburn: Many women experience heartburn (also known as indigestion or acid reflux) during the pregnancy. This is a burning sensation that usually extends from the bottom of the breastbone to the lower throat.

The greatly expanded uterus or womb exerts pressure on the stomach which in turn leads to the reflux of acid present in the stomach into the oesophagus or gullet to cause the burning sensation just alluded to.

Constipation: Constipation is a common problem during pregnancy. During pregnancy, the body produces more female hormones than usual. One of the hormones, progesterone, leads to a relaxation of the bowel muscles making them less able to move food and bodily waste along, causing constipation.

In the last months of pregnancy, the growing baby also exerts pressure on the bowels, which in turn leads to constipation.

Lower Back Pain: This is due among other factors to the increase in weight that goes with the pregnancy and the change of posture that comes about as a result of the pregnancy.

PREGNANCY COMPLICATIONS

Having outlined some of the signs and symptoms of a normal pregnancy, I shall now turn my attention to consider some of the complications, some of which can be serious, indeed, life-threatening, to both mother and child.

ECTOPIC PREGNANCY

The uterus is there to nourish a pregnancy. Unfortunately, in some instances, after fertilization has taken place, the zygote or the fertilized egg implants outside the lumen of the womb. This results in an ectopic pregnancy or a pregnancy that is "out of place". In about 95% of cases, ectopic pregnancies involve the fallopian tube.

Apart from the fallopian tube, the fertilized egg may also implant in the ovary, cervix or in the abdomen. Such areas are incapable of providing the needed space and nourishment required for the normal development of the pregnancy. As the fetus grows and expands, eventually the organ containing it bursts. This can lead to severe bleeding and a life-threatening situation to the would-be mother.

Signs and Symptoms: Symptoms of an ectopic pregnancy can be difficult to diagnose because they are similar to those of a normal early pregnancy— a missed period, breast tenderness, nausea, vomiting, etc.

The first real warning signs of an ectopic pregnancy are often pain or vaginal bleeding. Most women describe the pain as sharp and stabbing. It can be felt in the pelvis, abdomen and in some cases even in the shoulder or neck. (Blood built up from the ruptured ectopic pregnancy could irritate nerves supplying those areas.)

Apart from pain and bleeding, the following could also point to an ectopic pregnancy:

- vaginal spotting
- dizziness or fainting (caused by blood loss)
- low blood pressure (also caused by blood loss)
- lower back pain

Risk Factors: In theory any woman can be affected. The risk however is highest for women who are 35 years old and above and have had:

- a previous ectopic pregnancy
- previous surgery on a fallopian tube
- pelvic inflammatory disease (PID)

Treatment: Treatment of an ectopic pregnancy varies, depending on how medically stable the woman is and the size and location of the pregnancy.

Doctors may treat an early ectopic pregnancy by:

1. Injection: Medication could be injected to stop the further growth of the embryo.
2. Surgery: This is particularly the case in an emergency situation involving life-threatening bleeding.

MISCARRIAGE

Miscarriage is the loss of the baby during the earlier weeks of pregnancy. The World Health Organisation (WHO) defines it as being up to 23 weeks of the pregnancy and 500 grams in weight. There are variations in the period of time set by the WHO from country to country. This can vary from 20 weeks till up to 28 weeks of pregnancy.

Early miscarriage is mainly due to the fetus failing to develop normally. Later miscarriage on its part is more likely to be the result of the placenta not functioning properly or a weak cervix. Symptoms include bleeding, but this is not always the case and about half of all women who bleed in the early stages of pregnancy do not go on to miscarry.

PRE-ECLAMPSIA

Pre-eclampsia is a condition related to increased blood pressure and protein in the mother's urine. It typically starts after the 20th week of pregnancy. The causes are not entirely clear, but are thought to be related to defects in the placenta (after-birth).

Risk Factors: Some mothers are more at risk of developing pre-eclampsia. These include mothers with:

- a first pregnancy
- diabetes
- previously diagnosed hypertension
- multiple pregnancy (twins or triplets, etc.)
- a previous history of pre-eclampsia.
- a history of kidney disease.

Treatment: Regular blood pressure and urine checks will help detect pre-eclampsia. Once the condition is diagnosed, frequent monitoring of blood pressure, urinary protein excretion and weight become essential. If the condition worsens and the mother or baby or both is/are at risk, labour may be induced or a caesarean section performed.

GESTATIONAL DIABETES

Gestation diabetes is a condition in which women who have not been known to have diabetes before, exhibit high blood glucose levels during pregnancy.

As we saw earlier on, insulin is needed to transport sugar from the bloodstream to the cells.

In pregnancy, there is a higher demand on the pancreas to produce insulin. In some women, the pancreas is not able to meet the increased demand for insulin.

Risk Factors: These include obesity, women aged over 35 years as well as women with a previous history of gestational diabetes

Treatment: Treatment for gestational diabetes will depend on the severity of the diabetes. The goals of treatment are to keep blood glucose levels within normal limits during the duration of the pregnancy, and to ensure the well-being of mother and the developing baby.

- **Diet:** Mild forms can be treated with diet, in particular by decreasing the intake of simple sugars and fats.
- **Exercise**: Regular physical activity is sometimes used to keep blood sugar levels lower because contracting muscles help stimulate glucose transport.
- **Insulin**: When the above measures fail to keep blood glucose levels within an acceptable range, insulin injections are resorted to.

Gestational diabetes usually disappears following delivery though women who experience the condition have an increased risk of developing Type 2 Diabetes later in life.

BLEEDING

Bleeding during pregnancy could be scary and should be taken seriously. Fortunately such bleeding doesn't always have a serious underlying cause.

Bleeding during pregnancy could however have serious underlying causes. These may include:

- ectopic pregnancy
- threatened miscarriage
- placenta previa and
- placental abruption.

Placenta Previa: In this condition the placenta is fixed at a lower than usual position in the womb, and lies over the opening of the cervix. Placenta previa will often correct itself during pregnancy. In case it fails to do so and it leads to bleeding, doctors will assess the severity of the condition and decide on either emergency caesarean section or on monitoring the patient in hospital for a while.

Placental Abruption: In this case, the placenta has come away from the wall of the womb. It occurs usually from about 28 weeks onwards and usually causes sudden severe abdominal pain with some dark red bleeding or clots. It may necessitate in some cases an emergency caesarean section. If the symptoms are less severe, a short period of monitoring in hospital may be all that is required.

Chapter 22

Menopause

ⵉ

O ne day one of my patients consulted me to report a peculiar condition that had been plaguing her for a while.

The symptoms, she went on, included hot flushes that would suddenly descend on her. According to her, her body would in such moments feel very hot, as if in a hot oven. In such moments she would feel like pulling off her clothing, even if she happened to be walking on the street!

The hot sensation, she continued, could suddenly go to the other extreme, and she would experience a sensation of coldness. She would feel like she was freezing—indeed, as if she were living in the middle of a severe winter!

She also reported night sweats, sweats that were so extreme that her bedding became drenched in sweat! Partly as a result of the night sweats, she was forced to turn and turn in her sleep, something that was disturbing not only her sleep, but that of her husband as well.

"At times," she said, "my husband is so scared by my behaviour he thinks I may be going crazy!"

The symptoms displayed by my patient are among some of the typical ones associated with menopause.

What is Menopause?

In a previous chapter, I explained the menstrual cycle and its role in reproduction.

Every exciting game, it is said, must at some stage come to an end. The same is true of human life, at least in our present stage.

"Dust you are and to dust you shall return." Almighty God, having passed judgement on Adam and Eve, could in no way reverse the verdict.

If human life will have to come to an end, then a mechanism must be put into place to prevent the individual, who, as it were, is only on a transitional journey through the world, from bringing up offspring after a certain point in life.

Menopause in the strictest sense of the word is the permanent cessation of menstruation. A woman is generally considered to have reached menopause when she hasn't menstruated for twelve months. The time of onset of menopause differs from woman to woman. For most women it occurs between the ages of 40 and 56 years.

There is usually a transitional period, the pre-menopausal period. Again, this can differ from woman to woman. In some women it can last several years; in other women it can be a matter of just a few weeks. The pre-menopausal period is characterised by irregular menstruation.

For the majority of women the onset of menopause or the transition to that stage is uneventful. As in the case of the abovementioned patient, menopause can present symptoms that in some cases can be scary and burdensome.

It is important that women are educated on the matter, so that they do not behave like the woman I referred to at the beginning, who associated the symptoms of her condition to a possible spell cast on her by her rival.

SYMPTOMS

My patient has already described three typical symptoms of the condition, namely hot flushes, night sweats, and sleep disturbance.

Other symptoms are:

- dry skin, including drying of the genital organ
- thinning of the skin
- itching
- joint pains
- mood changes which can lead to irritability, anxiety, nervousness and depression
- fatigue (feeling tired all the time)
- weight gain

MANAGEMENT OF MENOPAUSE –RELATED SYMPTOMS

Hormone Replacement Therapy (HRT): Hormone Replacement Therapy (HRT) is an option for providing relief from symptoms of menopause. Since many problems associated with the menopause are believed to be due to reduced oestrogen levels, the main component of hormone replacement therapy (HRT) is oestrogen, although some preparation may include progesterone.

Because it replaces female hormones produced by the ovaries, hormone replacement therapy minimizes menopause symptoms such as night sweats, hot flushes, mood swings, genital dryness, etc.

One of the disadvantages of HRT therapy is that it is associated with a slightly increased risk of developing blot clots, ovarian cancer and breast cancer in some susceptible women over the age of 50.

Natural Remedies: Some women choose to avoid HRT and prefer to resort to natural remedies in the form of vitamins, herbs, soy, and dietary changes to help with the symptoms of menopause.

- **Remifemin**, obtained from Black cohosh, which is part of the buttercup family of plants, is purported to relieve symptoms of menopause—depression, night sweats, hot flashes, anxiety and irritability.
- **Phytoestrogens** or plant estrogens are natural compounds similar to oestrogen that help to alleviate a variety of menopausal symptoms.

Phytoestrogens are found in foods such as fruits, sprouts, red clover, yogurt, lentils and spinach.

PART 5

MEN'S HEALTH

Chapter 23

Benign Prostatic Hyperplasia (BPH)

The prostate gland is a chestnut-shaped organ found only in the male. It is located beneath the bladder and surrounds the urethra, the tube through which urine passes from the bladder into the penis. It plays an important role in the male reproductive system, producing the liquid that provides not only nutrients for sperm, but also protects and helps to drive them forward in the process of ejaculation.

In the young adult, the prostate gland weighs around 20g. As one grows old, the prostate gland tends to increase in size. Eventually it could grow to weigh as much as 150g. Often the condition is benign or non-cancerous and is referred to as benign prostatic hypertrophy (BPH).

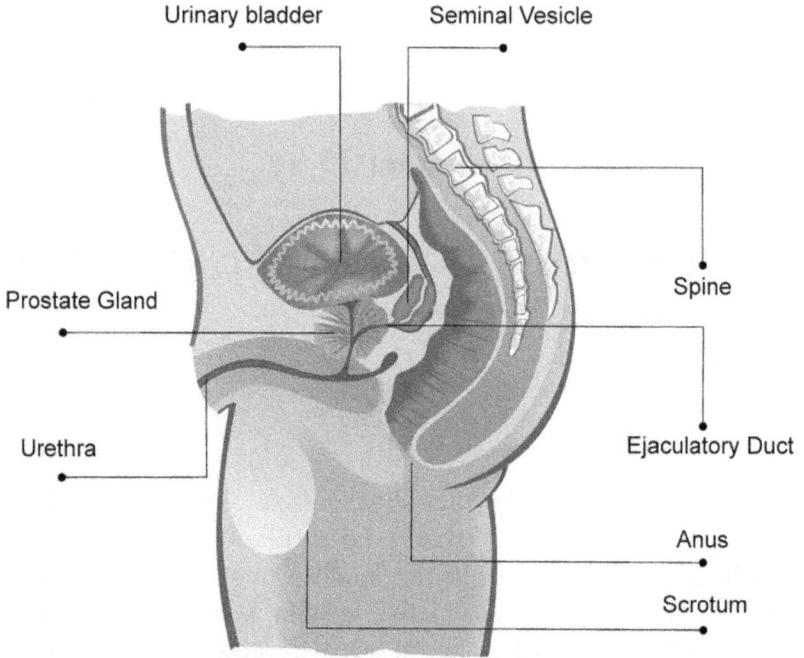

Position of the prostate gland in the body

SYMPTOMS

As the prostate grows, it constricts the urethra which in turn could lead to some of the symptoms listed below:

- Urinary frequency, i.e. the need to empty the bladder often, not only during the day but also at night, something which in turn could lead to sleep disturbance.
- Difficulty in starting the urine flow.
- Dribbling after urination.
- Decrease in the size and strength of the urine stream.

TREATMENT

- **Medication:** The medication in use either reduces the size of the enlarged prostate or relaxes the muscles in the prostate gland. Either way, the aim of therapy is an easing or elimination of the obstruction of urine through the urethra.
- **Surgery:** Surgery is resorted to where medication has not brought the desired effect. The standard surgical procedure is referred to as transurethral resection of the prostate gland (TURP). It involves the use of a device equipped with a small camera and a small sharp instrument which enables the surgeon to cut away excess prostate tissue.
- **Emergency Surgery in BPH**: BPH can sometimes lead to a medical emergency situation referred to as acute urinary retention. This is a situation whereby the enlarged prostate gland leads to a complete obstruction or blockage in the passage of urine to the outside. This usually necessitates surgical intervention whereby a cut is made on the lower abdominal wall and into the bladder. A catheter, suprapubic catheter, is then put in place to help drain the urine.

Chapter 24

Impotence /Erectile Dysfunction (ED)

∞

And God blessed them, and God said unto them, Be fruitful, and multiply, and replenish the earth, and subdue it: and have dominion over the fish of the sea, and over the fowl of the air, and over every living thing that moveth upon the earth. Genesis 1:28
And Adam knew Eve and they conceived Seth. Genesis 4:1

In an earlier chapter I mentioned that despite the general inclination of society to apportion blame to the woman when couples are infertile, medical science has established that the fault could equally lie in the man's court.

Before I move on further to consider the causes of male infertility I wish to clarify a point—impotence (erectile dysfunction) should not be confused with male infertility. Indeed, one can be potent, that is, be in a position to perform the role expected of him in a marriage relationship, and still be infertile.

As I mentioned earlier, it was the desire of Almighty God to co-operate with humankind in the multiplication of our race. To facilitate this, He placed at the disposal of both sexes not only the organs, but also the mechanisms needed to bring this about.

When, as a doctor, I sit down to ponder all the mechanisms at work in the body to facilitate the proper functioning of the male sexual organ, I just cannot help but wonder at the power and authority of the Divine.

Just like everything else created perfect by Almighty God, the normal functioning of the male sexual organ came to an end after Adam and Eve had disobeyed God. That brings me to the matter of erectile dysfunction.

I think an understanding of the mechanism at work in the male to ensure a proper erection is important to an understanding of erectile dysfunction, the situation when the mechanism, as it were, grinds either to a complete or partial stop.

Almighty God built the male sexual organ as two chambers. As a next step, He filled the chambers with a spongy tissue known as corpora canernosa, within which are muscles, fibrous tissues, spaces, veins, and arteries. He then wrapped the spongy chambers in a thick membrane called the tunica albuginea. To facilitate the communication of the rod-like object with the outside world, the Great Designer bored a tunnel through the underside of the organ to serve not only as a route for the sperm on their mission to fertilise the egg, but also as a passage for urine on its journey to the outside of the body.

Sensory and mental stimulation trigger the erection process. Several body parts work together to ensure it works. In the first place, the brain sends a message of sexual arousal through the nervous system to the male sexual organ. This message causes the muscles of the corpora cavernosa to relax. At the same time, the size of the artery, the vessel carrying blood from the heart to supply the organ, expands to twice its original size. As a result, the volume of blood it carries increases to about sixteen times compared to what it was before.

If only the matter would end there! But no, the Great Designer took further steps to ensure the desired effect was achieved, namely the stiffening and enlargement of the male sexual organ to facilitate sperm transport to the female. Consequently, simultaneous to the tremendous increase in the blood supply to the male sexual organ, the veins, the vessels responsible for transporting blood away from the penis, is blocked; blood is thus trapped and cannot escape.

The tunica albuginea, the thick wall wrapped around the corpora cavernosa, also plays an important role in helping to trap the blood and in so doing sustain the erection.

The Creator put the mechanism in place to ensure the process of erection reverses after a while. The process begins with the contraction of the muscles of the organ. This reduces the inflow of blood to the levels that persisted before the erection process. Simultaneously, the blockage on the walls of the veins lifts to allow outflow of blood.

CAUSES

Several factors can come into play to cause the dysfunction of the mechanism outlined above. These include the following:

- Diabetes—by adversely affecting the blood vessels of the body, diabetes negatively influences the mechanism of erection.
- Smoking. The effect of smoking could be compared to that of diabetes—smoking adversely affects the vessels.
- Alcohol Abuse—it does so mainly by adversely affecting the nerves.
- Spinal Cord and Brain injuries. From the mechanism of erection outlined above, one can easily understand why a brain or spinal cord injury could have an unfavourable effect on the erection mechanism.
- Diseases that affect the Nervous System: stroke, multiple sclerosis.
- Side effects of certain drugs, notable some blood pressure medication and anti-depressants.
- Effects of recreational drugs such as cocaine.
- Stress and mental disorder. Indeed, a certain degree of vitality in the individual is required for the system to function. We all know how we feel after we have spent eight, ten, twelve or sometimes more hours on our feet engaged in a very strenuous activity. Stress in this case does not apply only to physical stress; indeed,

emotional stress, even problems in the relationship, could, if only in the short term, negatively influence the system.
- Ageing. With increasing age comes increasing damage to the vessels of the body, including those that supply blood to the male genitalia. This in turn can lead to erectile dysfunction.

TREATMENT

In some cases, treating the underlying cause of the problem will lead to an improvement in the situation. Where that is not the case, my advice is that you contact your own doctor to discuss the best way forward. As I have all along stressed, we should not overlook the importance of prayer in all aspect of our health, including in this case, the sensitive issue of erectile dysfunction.

Chapter 25

Male Infertility

∞

Having considered the causes of erectile dysfunction, I shall now tackle male infertility in the broader sense. Indeed ED is only one factor among several possible causes of the condition.

For the male to be fertile several conditions need to be met:

- In the first place, the individual involved must be in a position to produce mature sperm.
- Next, that individual should be in a position not only to have an erection, but also to sustain it so as to be able to discharge the sperm into the female.
- The sperm should be in sufficient quantity and have the quality to be able to bring about fertilization.

Failure to meet any of the above conditions could lead to infertility.

CAUSES

Erectile Dysfunction—this has already been discussed above.

Testicular factors: there are situations where the testes, which can be described as a factory for the production of sperm, produce low quantity and/or poor quality sperm.

Following are some of the factors that can lead to such a situation:

- **Cryptorchidism**: During the time a male person is developing in his mother's womb, the testes first form in the stomach. In the course of time, they descend into the scrotum. Latest, by the time of birth, both testes should have done so. There are instances however when either one or both testes fail to do so. Within one year after birth, about 80% of the testes that had failed to descend do so retrospectively. Undescended testes are associated with reduced fertility. This is because sperm require a temperature lower than that found in the body to develop (the temperature in the scrotum is lower than that of the body).
- **Hydrocele**. I mentioned earlier the case of the resident in my little village carrying a huge hydrocele of the scrotum around the little settlement. A hydrocele testis can adversely affect the production of sperm.
- **Hormonal Problems**. Deficiency of the male hormone, testosterone, can lead to a decrease in sperm production which in turn can lead to reduced fertility.
- **Smoking** has been shown to reduce both sperm count and sperm motility.
- **Alcohol**. Excessive intake of alcohol can lead to a low sperm count and have a detrimental effect on male fertility.
- **Stress, emotional or physical, can each or in combination cause** low sperm count, which in turn can lead to reduced fertility.

TREATMENT

As in the case of erectile dysfunction, treating the underlying cause of male infertility may lead to a reversal of the situation. Should the condition persist, you should contact your doctor to discuss the best way forward.

PART 6
CANCER

Chapter 26

General Symptoms, Diagnosis &
Treatment of Cancer

C ancer is indeed a common word which among other things conjures up fear and apprehension in many—and not without cause. Cancer can indeed bring about death—our physical death.

Now since this book is meant principally for Christians, I want to pause for a moment to reflect on the issue of cancer, based on Scripture.

In Romans 6:23 we read:

For the wages of sin is death; but the gift of God is eternal life through Jesus Christ our Lord.

I believe it is not our physical death Apostle Paul is referring to here, but rather spiritual death, the eternal separation from the King of Kings and Lord of Lords.

Now we fear cancer because it has the potential to lead to death—physical death. The question to ponder here is: do we fear sin the same way that we fear cancer? Do we fear sin, yes, flee from sin in the same way we would should we spot cancer, that general, dreadful foe, coming our way?

What, then, is cancer?

Many of us have indeed heard the word *cancer*. It is when it comes to the details, what really lies behind the term, that the problem begins.

I will at this stage attempt to provide an explanation in a manner that, hopefully, everyone can understand.

Almighty God made our bodies of cells. The cell indeed is the basic unit, or building block, of life. All living things are made up of one or more cells. Organisms may exist as single cells (unicellular), or, like ourselves, as a group of cells working together, (multicellular).

The cells in our body are constantly undergoing wear, tear and death. For life to continue, cells must be able to divide or replicate to replace the dead ones. Usually the cells divide in a controlled manner.

The parent cell, in a process known as mitosis, divides into two so-called daughter cells. Each daughter cell after a while becomes a parent cell that in turn divides into two daughter cells; and so on, and on, the process continues, so long as life continues. In cancer, this control mechanism has gone out of control. Put in a simple way, cancer cells, the moment they begin to divide, continue unabated to divide, divide and divide.

Will you permit me, dear reader, to reflect on the matter for a while? I do indeed recognise in the tendency of cancer cells to divide in an uncontrolled manner a parallel with how sin can also spread uncontrollably.

Let us for example consider the issue between King David and Bathsheba, the wife of Uriah. For the sake of space, I am not going to reproduce the whole text here. The story is recorded in 2 Samuel 11.

It all began when David lusted after Bathsheba in his heart; next, he moved on to commit adultery and, finally, murder. In the end, therefore, it brought misery to him and his household.

We must, indeed, guard against sinful tendencies, for, like cancer cells, sin can indeed spread in an uncontrollable fashion.

Back to the cancer cells. What makes cancer cells a nuisance to the body is the fact that they are incapable of performing the functions of the original cell from which they developed. Let us take white blood cells as an example.

The white blood cells, as we saw earlier, are there to defend the body against outside invaders. White blood cells that have turned cancerous, known also as leukaemia cells, whilst swimming in abundance in the liquid part of the blood (plasma) are, to put it bluntly, good for nothing—just good for nothing!

Yet another feature of cancer cells—they can, without exaggeration, be described as insatiable gluttons! Always hungry for food, they voraciously consume a considerable portion of whatever nutrients their poor victims are able to supply to their bodies.

If only the cancer cells would restrict themselves to the organ in which they developed. Indeed, if only, for example, cancer cells that have developed in the pancreas would confine their destructive activities to that organ only.

It is said that the moment you offer some human beings one centimetre, they go on to demand one metre. The same thing can be said of the cancer cells. For example, cancer cells of the pancreas would sooner rather than later leave the walls of the pancreas and begin to infiltrate, penetrate and invade neighbouring tissues and organs.

One might assume that would be the end of the matter, but no! Ultimately, cancer cells of the pancreas could move to settle in the brain, the liver, and the bones! How did they get there, one might wonder? Well, the answer is simple—through the bloodstream and the lymphatic system.

One might imagine that cancer cells, on arrival in their new hosts, would stay quiet and enjoy the kind hospitality accorded them. That unfortunately is seldom the case. On the contrary, no sooner have they settled into their new environment than they resume their malicious activity of uncontrolled division.

Soon, instead of brain cells growing in the skull of the victim, pancreas cells will be doing so as well.

Cancer cells, as it were, will be changing the destiny of the target organ, just the same way that sin can change the destiny of those it rules over.

GENERAL SYMPTOMS OF CANCER

Different types of cancer produce different symptoms, depending on the organ involved. There are however symptoms that most cancers share in common. Here are a few of them:

- **Persistent Fatigue (feeling tired all the time).** Fatigue is not unique to cancer. Several other factors—stress, anaemia, malnutrition, lack of vitamins, chronic infectious diseases such as HIV etc.—could also lead to the condition.

    Still, one should have cancer in mind, especially in case fatigue persists over a considerable period of time.
- **Weight Loss.** If you happen to be overweight and have actively contributed to a reduction in weight, more grease to your elbow! If, on the other hand, you have all of a sudden, inadvertently, lost a substantial amount of weight, you are advised to have a health check to rule out cancer and other diseases associated with weight loss.
- **Loss of Appetite;** should it linger on for a while, could point to various kinds of diseases including cancer.
- **Pain.** Several conditions can cause pain to the body. In cancer, pain is usually not an early sign of the disease. Instead, it is generally associated with advanced stages of the disease, especially at the stage when it has gained in size or spread to other parts of the body, in particular the bone.
- **Fever.** Earlier in my discourse I dealt with fever and cited the various conditions that can lead to fever. Fever, usually, is a transitional condition. Should the condition however persist for long, it could be a sign of cancer, especially blood cancer (leukaemia) or cancer that has spread to other parts of the body.
- **Night sweats.** Unexplained sweating in the night could be due to several conditions—menopause, infections, diabetes, but also cancer (such as leukaemia).

GENERAL PRINCIPLES OF CANCER DIAGNOSIS

There are several general principles applied by medical science in cancer diagnosis.One of the most important tools is screening.

Screening: Cancer cells are normal body cells gone astray. The most effective way to contain them is to fight them at the very early stage of development, long before they are able to spread to neighbouring as well as distant organs.

Now, how can you and I, ordinary human beings with limited resources at our disposal, become aware that at any time of our existence, some of our cells, cells that until then have dutifully served us, have all of the sudden turned into cancer cells poised to destroy us?

Screening is the only effective tool available to medical science that has the means of detecting the problem—in other words, that can detect and identify the presence of cancer cells in our body as early as possible. It enables the doctor to detect cancer cells in order to come to a decision to take the appropriate action to curtail or eradicate them. It is indeed true that as far as the treatment of cancer goes, time is of the greatest essence. Screening aims to find, attack and destroy cancer cells as early as possible before they are able to destroy their victim.

GENERAL PRICIPLES OF CANCER TREATMENT

Before I consider a few selected cases of cancers in detail, I want to consider the general principles behind the treatment of cancer.

As I mentioned earlier, cancer basically is uncontrolled cell division that leads to the development of tumours.

- **Surgery**: Removal of the tumour, especially in the early stages, will help prevent the spread to other organs. In an advanced stage, a stage when cancer has spread to other parts of the body, surgery may still be needed especially if the growth is pressing on neighbouring organs thereby preventing the organs involved from performing their functions.

  For example, if cancer is compressing the gullet, preventing the victim from swallowing, surgery could be performed to alleviate the situation.

- **Radiation Therapy:** This involves the use of high-energy x-rays or other types of radiation to kill cancer cells or keep them from growing.
- **Chemotherapy**: In Chemotherapy, the patient is prescribed drugs with the goal of stopping the growth of cancer cells either by killing them or preventing them from dividing.

One form of the three types of therapy outlined here does not exclude the other. In other words, the said types of therapy can be combined in various ways with the goal of achieving the best possible results.

I will now move on to consider a few common cancers in some detail.

Chapter 27

BREAST CANCER

༄

A lthough men can develop breast cancer, the disease is about a hundred times more common in women than in men.

When we come to consider that the most potent attribute given to women by Almighty God to attract the male has also become a source of her woes, we realise that we do indeed live on a fallen planet! For the follower of Our Lord and Saviour Jesus Christ, the outlook is not as bleak as it may seem, for we are indeed overcomers through Him who overcame sin, Satan and death on the cross of Calvary.

RISK FACTORS

Medical science has identified several risk factors in the development of breast cancer. Some can be classified as low risks, others as high. I will only name a few. It must be said that as in several aspects of medical practice, there is not a general consensus among the experts regarding how much weight should be given to the various risk factors.

Genetics: It has been observed that the condition has the tendency to occur in families. For example, it has been observed that if a mother suffered from the condition, some of her daughters also may have gone on to suffer from the condition. That is a conclusion that has been reached by medical science based on a study of several cases of the condition. We cannot run away from that fact.

Now, what attitude should Christians who happen to belong to such a family adopt? Before I attempt an answer, I want us to look at Psalm 23:1 as well as Psalm 23:4

> *The LORD is my shepherd; I shall not want. Psalm 23:1*
> *Yea, though I walk through the valley of the shadow of death, I will fear no evil: for thou art with me; thy rod and thy staff they comfort me. Psalm 23:4*

What do we learn from David in Psalm 23?

David, through Divine Inspiration, is telling the Church that the Lord is our Shepherd, so we shall not want, or be in need of anything.

He goes on to state that even though we walk through the valley of the shadow of death, with cancer staring us in the face, we need not fear evil.

Based on the above, my advice to such an individual is do not panic! You should nevertheless carry on with frequent screenings/checks and leave the rest to the Lord.

I pray for the Lord to increase your faith so that you do not, out of desperation, go to the extent of undergoing what is termed prophylactic breast amputation, whereby you will sign for the doctors to remove your healthy breasts out of fear that they may develop cancer later in life.

In this case also, I want to make it clear that I am not trying to play the big judge. No, I am not condemning those individuals who out of concern undergo such procedure. I am only praying that we could in such a situation, be able to develop sufficient faith to place our destiny in the hands of the Lord. As my driving school teacher used to say, death becomes our companion the moment we get behind the wheel of our vehicle and set the vehicle rolling. Do we as a result decide never to travel in a vehicle?

Personal History of Breast Cancer: A woman who has had cancer in one breast has an increased risk of developing a new cancer in the other breast or in another part of the same breast. This is different from a recurrence (return) of the first cancer.

Age at Childbirth: Studies have shown that women who happened to give birth to their first child at an older age or who have never given birth run the risk of developing the condition.

Contraceptive Pill: Women who take the contraceptive pill have been observed to tend to develop breast cancer as compared to women who are not on the pill.

Being overweight or obese: Being overweight or obese has been found to increase the risk of breast cancer, especially after menopause.

Alcohol: the use of alcohol increases the risk in the development of various cancers, including breast cancer. The rule seems to be the more alcohol one drinks the greater the risk of cancer.

Breastfeeding: Some studies suggest that breastfeeding may slightly lower breast cancer risk, especially if breastfeeding is continued for a period of about eighteen to twenty-four months.

There are a few other risk factors in the literature which are not touched on here. Those interested in learning more may consult the relevant literature. For the sake of our current discussion, I consider the points already touched on to be sufficient.

DIAGNOSIS

Self-Examination: In breast cancer, self-examination by a woman if properly done can be an invaluable screening method.

Health experts advise women to begin self-examining their breast by the age of twenty years. In this connection the experts recommend that women examine themselves about a week after the first day of their period, at a time when the breasts are no longer swollen and tender due to hormonal fluctuations. Any new changes should be reported to a doctor or a health professional, as the case may be. Of course, this recommendation can apply only to women living in areas where there is easy access to medical care. For women living in remote areas of our planet, like the remote African village where my eyes first saw the light of day, matters are not that straightforward.

What should a woman look out for on self-examining her breasts?

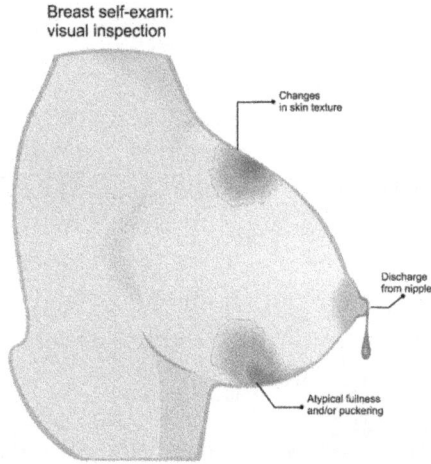

Breast self-exam:
visual inspection

Changes
in skin texture

Discharge
from nipple

Atypical fullness
and/or puckering

Changes in breast cancer

- Changes in the look or feel of the skin over the breast, especially if it looks dimpled, puckered or like orange peel.
- A lump, or a thickening or bumpy area in the breast or armpit, which is absent from the other breast or armpit.
- A discharge from the nipple that is new and which is not milk.
- More than the ordinary discomfort or pain in one breast, particularly if it refuses to go away after several days.
- Bleeding from the nipple.
- Any changes in the nipple position, like when it appears to be pulled up or pointing differently.
- A rash on or around the nipple.
- Moist red areas on the nipple that do not heal easily.

- A breast that feels warm to touch, much warmer than the other breast. It could be a sign of inflammatory breast cancer.

Clinical Breast Examination: Apart from self-examination, it is recommended that women above the age of twenty undergo clinical breast examination once a year through a nurse, a family doctor or a gynaecologist as the case may be. (In this case also it is a matter of access to corresponding medical care.)

Mammogram: This can be described as a breast x-ray. It is regarded as the gold standard for breast cancer screening and early detection. In some advanced societies, it is recommended that women above the age of 40 years have an annual mammogram. Mammograms are credited to help detect 85 to 90 per cent of all breast cancers, even those that are too small to be felt during manual examination.

TREATMENT

Treatment for breast cancer is based on the general principles of cancer treatment outlined above.

Surgery: Surgery could be in the form of:

- **Lumpectomy:** which involves the removal of the tumour and a small amount of normal tissue around it.
- **Partial mastectomy**: removal of the part of the breast that has cancer and some normal tissue around it.
- **Total mastectomy:** this type of surgery is resorted to in an advanced stage of cancer, when cancer might already have spread to other parts of the body. This involves complete removal of the breast and surrounding tissue, including lymph nodes.

Surgery could be followed by one or more of the following:

- Radiation therapy
- Chemotherapy
- Hormone therapy. It is believed that hormones produced in the body sustain the growth of cancer cells. The aim of hormone therapy is to block the effect of such hormones on the growth of the breast cancer cells.

Chapter 28

Cervical Cancer

CD

C ervical cancer is cancer affecting the cervix or the neck of the uterus (womb).

CAUSES

Medical science cannot exactly pinpoint the cause of cervical cancer. However, it has been established that the condition is strongly associated with Human Papilloma Virus (HPV)

RISK FACTORS

There are several risk factors. This book will touch on some of them. What I said about breast cancer is also true here—those wanting to know more are advised to read the relevant literature.

Human Papilloma Virus: HPV infection is one of the most significant risk factors in cervical cancer. This does not imply that every HPV infection will lead to cervical cancer. There are said to be approximately forty-six different kinds of HPV. Of the number only a few lead to the development of cancer. (As you may recall, one strain of the virus causes genital warts.)

Sexual behaviour: As we saw above, the Human Papilloma Virus is sexually transmitted. The development of cervical cancer is thus strongly correlated with sexual behaviour.

It is generally agreed that a woman has a higher risk of developing cervical cancer if she:

- Has had multiple sexual partners.
- Began having sexual relations early. By that the literature generally speaks of sexual contact before the age of 18 years.
- Has sex with partners who themselves have many partners.

The risks associated with sexual behaviour come down, in the end, to the risk of HPV infection. In this connection emphasis needs to be placed on the number of sexual partners. The more sexual partners one has, the more likely is the chance of contracting an HPV infection which could eventually develop into cervical cancer. For example, a 17-year-old who stays with the same faithful partner, who in turn remains faithful to her, is less likely to be infected by HPV and go on to develop cervical cancer, than the case of a 20-year-old who has multiple partners who, on their part, also boast of multiple partners.

Smoking: Women who smoke are about twice as likely to develop cervical cancer as women who do not. The more a woman smokes—and the longer she has been smoking—the greater the risk.

Weakened immune system: As I mentioned earlier, a weakened immune system generally impairs the body's ability to fight infections and other diseases, including cancer, in this case cervical cancer.

SYMPTOMS

In its early stage, cervical cancer may not cause noticeable signs or symptoms. Later signs of cervical cancer include:

- **Abnormal genital bleeding**. Genital bleeding is however not unique for cervical cancer—other conditions could be present with similar symptoms.
- **Unusual vaginal discharge**. It may be foul smelling, watery, thick, or contain mucus. This is also not unique for cervical cancer.
- **Pelvic pain.** This can be mild or severe and can range from a dull ache to a sharp pain. It can persist for hours.
- **Pain and or bleeding after or during sexual intercourse**.

DIAGNOSIS

- Clinical Examination.
- Smear test (Pap smear). This involves scraping cells off the cervix and smearing them onto a glass slide and analysing them under a microscope for abnormality.
- Coloscopy. In coloscopy, a device known as a coloscope is used to view and examine the surface of the cervix for signs of abnormality. This also allows for the taking of a biopsy for further examination.

TREATMENT

In this case the general principles of cancer therapy also apply.

SURGERY: This may involve the following:

- **Conization**: This procedure involves the removal of a cone-shaped piece of tissue from the cervix and cervical canal.
- **Cryosurgery**: In this type of treatment an instrument is used to freeze and destroy the cancer cells (abnormal tissue).

- **Laser Surgery**: In this procedure a laser beam, a narrow beam of intense light, is applied like a knife to cut out and remove the tumour.

The above three methods are only used in cases where the tumour is discovered in the very early stages, at a time when it is confined only to the cervix.

- **Hysterectomy**: The term stands for the complete removal of the womb. This method is applied in cases where the cancer has already reached an advanced stage. There are two forms of the procedure:
- **Total hysterectomy**, which involves the removal of the uterus and cervix
- **Radical hysterectomy**, which involves not only the removal of the entire womb, but also the ovaries, fallopian tubes and surrounding lymph nodes.

Chapter 29

Cancer of the Womb (Endometrial Cancer)

∞

In the previous section we dealt with cancer of the cervix. As we learnt, this is cancer that affects the neck of the womb. I will now move on to consider cancer of the womb proper.

The hollow of the womb is lined by a layer of cells known as endometrium. As in the case of almost every cell of the body, cancer cells can develop from the cells of the endometrium.

Endometrial cancer is the fourth most common cancer that affects women, after breast, lung and colon cancer. It becomes more common after menopause.

RISK FACTORS

As in cervical cancer, it is not exactly known what causes cancer of the womb. Certain factors have however been observed to increase the risk. These include the following:

- Women who have never been pregnant: Studies have shown that women who have never given birth have a higher risk of developing the condition. Conversely the risk is lower in women who have had children.

- Obesity: Overweight or obese women are generally more likely to develop womb cancer than women of a normal weight.
- Age: Cancer of the womb becomes more common after menopause.
- Alcohol: Some studies have shown that women who drink considerable amounts of alcohol regularly have an increased risk of womb cancer compared to women who do not drink at all.

DIAGNOSIS

- **Clinical examination**.
  Depending on the medical facilities available, the clinical examination could be followed by one or more of the tests outlined below:
- **Biopsy**: As we saw earlier on, this involves the removal of tissue from the womb for further examination.
- **Hysteroscopy**: Where available, a device known as a hysteroscope can be used to view the inside of the womb. In the process a biopsy is taken.
- **Ultrasound scan**.

THERAPY

Surgery is one of the effective options to treat cancer of the womb. There are different types of surgeries that may be used, depending on the patient's condition. One of the common surgical procedures is total hysterectomy. This involves the complete removal of the womb, including the cervix.

Depending on the type of cancer, the stage of disease and the extent to which the cancer has spread, radiotherapy, hormone therapy and chemotherapy may also be resorted to, either in isolation or in combination with surgery.

Chapter 30

Lung Cancer

∞

L ike all organs of the body, the lung cells can also develop into cancer cells. The lung happens also to be a common site for the spread of cancers that have developed elsewhere in the body.

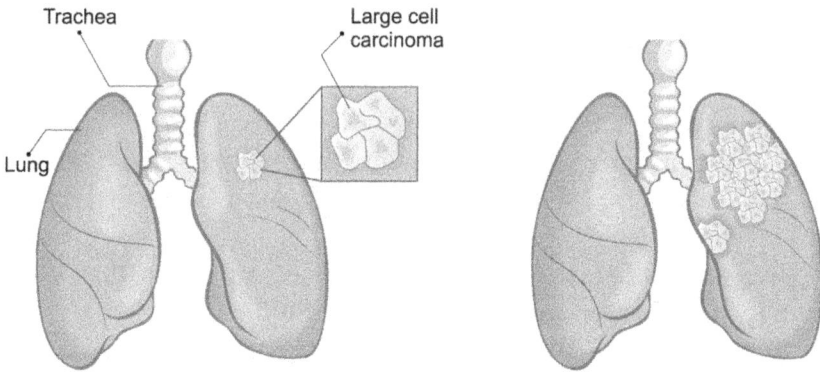

Lung Cancer

RISK FACTORS

- **Smoking**: The main risk factor in the development of lung cancer is cigarette smoking. It is true that there are instances when non-smokers have developed lung cancer. In the overwhelming number of cases (about nine out of ten), however, smokers are affected, whereas cigarette smokers are more at risk compared to pipe and cigar smokers.
- **Passive smoking:** Passive smoking, that is, the inhalation or breathing in of tobacco/cigarette smoke coming from other smokers, does increase the risk for the development of lung cancer, though this risk is much less than that for the active smoker.

In this connection, it is very encouraging that in several countries laws have been put in place to ban smoking in public places. It is hoped that those countries that have not done so, will sooner rather than later follow suit.

Other factors that increase the risk for the development of lung cancer are:

- **Asbetos**. Asbestos is the name given to a group of minerals that occur naturally in the environment as bundles of fibres. Individuals exposed to such fibres have an increased risk of developing lung cancer.
- **Radon gas.** Radon is a naturally occurring gas that seeps out of the ground in certain places. Studies have shown that individuals who are exposed to high concentrations of radon for a considerable period of time have an increased risk of developing lung cancer.
- **Air pollution**. Air pollution from vehicles, industry, and power plants, etc. is thought to have a small but significant increase in a person's lung cancer risk.

SYMPTOMS

As in the case of several forms of cancer, lung cancer may not cause any symptoms in the initial stages. As the disease advances, the following symptoms may become apparent:

- Shortness of breath
- Persistent coughing
- Coughing up blood
- Wheezing
- Chest pain

It must be said that the above symptoms are not exclusive for lung cancer. For example, lung tuberculosis can also lead to persistent coughing, and coughing of blood. Similarly, asthma may lead to shortness of breath and wheezing.

If, however, the symptoms appear in a person who has a long history of smoking and are accompanied by the other general cancer symptoms touched on earlier, one should suspect lung cancer.

DIAGNOSIS

- Clinical examination
- **X-ray**: Chest x-ray is the most common first diagnostic step.
- **CT-scan**: This can help not only to establish the primary tumour, but also to reveal the spread of the disease.
- **MRI-scan**.
- **Sputum cytology**: This involves the examination of the sputum of the affected person for evidence of cancer cells.
- **Bronchoscopy**: Where available, a device known as a bronchoscope is used to view the airways for signs of cancer. In the process a biopsy is taken for further examination.

TREATMENT

As in the majority of cancers, treatment involves surgery, radiotherapy and chemotherapy. These may be offered alone or in combination, depending on the type of cancer in question (there are two main types, non-small-cell lung cancer or small-cell lung cancer), how well the patient is and also the extent to which cancer has spread to other parts of the body.

Chapter 31

Prostate Cancer

∞

Earlier on, I dealt with benign prostate hyperplasia(BPH) and the symptoms associated with it. I will now turn my attention to cancer of the prostate gland.

CAUSES

Medical science cannot exactly pinpoint the causes.

RISK FACTORS

The following are some of the common risk factors linked with the condition:

- **Age**: It has been said that prostate cancer is a disease of old age. Men aged below 50 years have a low risk of developing the condition. The risk increases considerably after that age. It's estimated that around 80% of men in their 80s will have prostate cancer.
- **Ethnic background**: It has been observed that men of African descent are more likely to be affected than men of European and Asian descent.

- **Family history**: It has also been observed that men whose close relatives—father, brother, grandfather—have had the condition are slightly more likely to develop it themselves.

SYMPTOMS

The symptoms of prostate cancer can be similar to that occurring in BPH. They may include the following:

- Urinating frequently.
- Difficult or painful urination or ejaculation.
- Delay or hesitancy before urinating.
- A feeling that the bladder has not completely emptied.
- Blood in urine or semen.
- Disturbed sleep because of the need to empty the bladder at night.

DIAGNOSIS

Prostate-specific antigen (PSA) test: The main test for prostate cancer is the PSA test. PSA is a substance found in the blood of men. A rise of PSA above a certain value is a possible indication of prostate cancer. There is some current concern, however, about the accuracy of the PSA test and its usefulness. Some studies have shown that

- Up to 20% of men who do have prostate cancer will not have a raised PSA level;
- Over 65% of men with a raised PSA level will not have cancer since PSA levels tend to rise in all men as they get older.

Clinical Examination: The next step in confirming a diagnosis of prostate cancer is by way of clinical examination, specifically, by way of digital rectal examination (DRE). This involves the examiner inserting a finger in the rectum (back passage). The rectum is close to the prostate gland, a fact which enables the examiner to feel it. Usually the surface of the gland feels smooth to touch. Prostate cancer can cause the gland to become hard and bumpy. An experienced examiner will notice the difference and suspect cancer.

Biopsy: Cancer is usually established by taking a piece of tissue and examining it under the microscope.

Ultra Sound: Where available, the prostate gland can be examined with a type of ultrasound called transrectal ultrasonography. This is inserted into the rectum (back passage) to the nearby prostate.

MRI-Scan: MRI scans can create a clear picture of the prostate gland.

CT Scan: Tumors can better be seen with CT-Scans than with an ordinary X-ray

TREATMENT

If diagnosed early, treatment can be quite successful. The key decision in prostate cancer is whether or not to treat at all. In many older men, the cancer progresses so slowly that surgery and other treatments may cause more harm than good.

However, for those whose cancer is more aggressive, either already spreading or liable to spread beyond the prostate, surgery is usually the first option. Surgery involves the removal of the gland (prostatectomy) together with surrounding lymph nodes.

Surgery may lead to nerve damage, which in turn may lead to erection as well as urinary problems.

Chapter 32

Skin Cancer

∞

CAUSE

The main cause of skin cancer is overexposure to the sun's harmful ultraviolet (UV) rays.

OTHER RISK FACTORS

People with fair skin :Statistics have shown that the light-skinned individual is more vulnerable to develop the condition. It must be stressed that having a light skin alone is not an all-determining factor. What may have been observed to aggravate the situation is an over-exposure of the skin to ultra-violet rays, such as occurs during sunbathing.

Family history: People with a family history of melanoma have roughly double the risk of developing the disease compared to people without a family history

TYPES OF SKIN CANCER

BASAL CELL CARCINOMA: This is the most common type of skin cancer. It affects the basal cells. These are found within the top layer of skin. It is a slow- growing cancer and does not usually metastasize or spread to other parts of the body. Basal cell carcinoma affects all sun exposed areas of the body

Symptoms

It may appear as a small painless lump, brownish-grey in colour. It may develop a central depression with rolled edges.

SQUAMOUS CELL CARCINOMA: This type of skin cancer usually affects the face.

Symptoms

The main symptom is an area of thickened, scaly skin. This may develop into a painless, hard lump, reddish brown in colour with an irregular edge. The lump could develop into an ulcer which won't heal.

The above-named types of skin cancer are known as non-melanoma skin cancer to differentiate them from melanoma.

MELANOMA SKIN CANCER: Melanoma of the skin is related to the common mole. It is the most aggressive form of skin cancer and can occur anywhere on the body. It affects the melanin cells, the cells which produce the skin's colouring. If not identified and treated early, it can spread to affect the liver, lungs or brain.

Symptoms:

The main symptoms are: a quick-growing, irregular, dark-coloured spot on previously normal skin or on an existing mole that changes size, colour, develops irregular edges, bleeds, itches, crusts or reddens.

DIAGNOSIS

- **Clinical examination**: The condition might be suspected as a result of the changes outlined above.
- **Biopsy**: Any potential melanoma requires a surgical biopsy, also known as excisional biopsy, in which the entire growth is removed. The sample is then studied under a microscope to determine whether cancer cells are present.

TREATMENT OF SKIN CANCER

NON-MELANOMA:

- **Surgery**: Non-melanoma skin cancers are usually treated by a common operation to simply cut out the affected area under local anaesthetic.
- **Cryosurgery**: Another method used on smaller cancers is cryosurgery, in which liquid nitrogen is applied to the tumour to freeze it and kill the cells. The tumor will simply wither and drop off once warmed up.
- **Photodynamic therapy**: A so-called 'photodynamic therapy' is applied to treat some cases of basal cell carcinoma. This involves the use of a cream to sensitise the tumour. It is then exposed to high intensities of light to destroy it.

MELANOMA:

Treatment for melanoma depends on the extent of the disease, the patient's age and general health, and other factors.

Apart from the three general forms of cancer treatment outlined earlier, namely surgery, radiation therapy, chemotherapy, a fourth type, biological therapy, may be applied.

Biological therapy, making use of special proteins known as interferon, is resorted to especially in cases where cancer has spread to other parts of the body or in patients where there is a high risk of the cancer returning. Interferon acts to stimulate immune cells into attacking melanoma cells more aggressively.

PART 7

MENTAL HEALTH ISSUES

E arlier I stressed that, as Christians we will be spared many of the mental health problems that plague the world if we would adhere to the teaching of our blessed Lord.

In this section I will explain how medical science views some of the common disturbances that may affect the mind and how it attempts to cure them.

I have stressed all along that we should, as Christians, seek medical help when things go wrong in our body. When it comes to the area of mental health, however, I personally am sceptical about the ability of conventional medicine to provide an effective cure in several instances of mental illness.

How, for example, can tablets effectively help in a situation where a mental health disturbance, for example depression, has arisen as a result of a troubled marriage, say, as result of the unfaithfulness of one partner in a relationship?

Anti-depressants may, perhaps, provide temporal relief. In the long run, however, it is obvious that it is the root cause of the problem that needs to be tackled, not the symptoms. Having said that by way of introduction, I shall now move on to consider some of the mental health issues that plague us by dint of our fallen nature.

Chapter 33

Anxiety & Depression

∞

ANXIETY

A nxiety is a troubled state of mind characterised by uneasiness and apprehension—an almost permanent feeling of fear, worry as well as a feeling of being weighed down with care and concern, especially for the future.

Everyone experiences a certain degree of anxiety at some stage in life. I have in mind the football player or fan whose team is engaged in a penalty shoot out to decide the outcome of a crucial match. The heart as a result of the tense situation could start racing, the muscles could begin shaking involuntarily, sweat could break out to soak our clothes, etc.

Our team could end up losing the match. That could lead, in the short term, to disappointment, even bitter disappointment. That in turn could even lead to a sleepless night. That is a natural human reaction to a distressing situation.

The problem begins when anxiety, as it were, becomes an almost permanent guest in our home—when we begin to develop an excessive, uncontrollable and often irrational worry about everyday things, disproportionate to the actual source of worry. At this stage medical science speaks of generalised anxiety disorder.

CAUSES

The following are some of the factors identified by medical science as possible causes of anxiety.

- **Genes**: The fact that some tend to be more anxious than others has led medical science to conclude that it could have something to do with the genes we inherited from our parents. I personally take this explanation with a pinch of salt. As I mentioned earlier, there is the tendency these days to apportion our genes blame for several of the medical problems that confront us. I am inclined to think that an increased tendency to become anxious has more to do with our upbringing than our genes. Parents who tend to be anxious about many things may bring up their children in such a way as to impart that tendency on them. You may not see eye to eye with me on this matter. What we as Christians can agree upon, however, is that we are called upon to bring our cares and worries, no matter the cause, to the feet of the Cross of our loving Saviour.
- **Circumstances**: Our circumstances may lead to anxiety. For example, the threat of job loss, of deportation, of repossession of our homes, etc., may lead to anxiety.
- **Drugs**: The so-called recreational drugs like amphetamines, lysergic acid diethylamide, abbreviated LSD or ecstasy can lead to anxiety after their so-called "pleasurable effects" have subsided.

SYMPTOMS

The example about the penalty shoot-out touched on some of the symptoms associated with anxiety. These include the following:

- Feeling worried all the time
- Tiredness

- Irritability
- Sleep disturbance
- Difficulty concentrating
- Racing heartbeat
- Sweating
- Muscle tension and pains
- Shaking
- Feeling dizzy or faint

PANIC

This is a special form of anxiety and involves sudden and unexpected episodes of intense anxiety. Panic attacks share some of the symptoms of anxiety, e.g. accelerated heart rate, shaking, sweating, feeling dizzy, etc., though the said symptoms are experienced more intensely by the affected person.

DEPRESSION

Anxiety and depression are related in the sense that anxiety leads to depression. Anxiety is short-lived. Anxiety, should it persist for a long while, ends up in depression.

The state of mind of the depressed person is characterized among other things by feelings of sadness, gloom, despair, low self-esteem, self-reproach and discouragement.

The following are some of the life events that can lead to depression:

- **Bereavement**: Death of a family member, friend, or pet. Indeed, the death of a pet can lead to depression in some individuals.
- **Breakdown of relationships:** This can lead to depression not only in the affected individuals themselves but may also lead to depression in their children. (Yet another reason why the Church

213

should do all it can to prevent Christian marriages from breaking down.)

- **Birth of a child (postnatal depression):** What is usually regarded as a happy event can, unfortunately, lead to depression in some mothers.
- **Stressful situations**: Poverty, homelessness, job loss, violence in the family, constant relationship problems, etc. could also lead to depression.

FORMS OF DEPRESSION

Depression can come in various forms:

- **Major Depression**: Also known as unipolar depression, major depression could be intense and short-lived.
- **Dysthymia**: Also known as chronic depression, this type of depression, though less severe, is long-lasting.
- **Bipolar Disorder**: Bipolar disorder is characterized by periods of major depression alternating or combined with periods of mania. In mania the affected person experiences abnormally high moods and extreme bursts of unusual activity or energy. So, a person suffering a bipolar disorder feels down one day and extremely happy the next.

SYMPTOMS

A person suffering from depression may lose interest in life, a situation that could in turn lead to suicidal thoughts, attempts or in the worst case scenario, suicide.

Other symptoms are:

- Feeling of worthlessness

- Feeling of hopelessness
- Feeling of pessimism
- Feeling of guilt
- Finding it harder to make decisions
- Not coping with things that used to be manageable
- Exhaustion
- Feeling restless and agitated
- Loss of appetite and weight
- Sleeping difficulty

In short, as far as the depressed person is concerned, everything is gloom, gloom, gloom. He or she, as it were, considers him or herself as entrapped in a dark tunnel or locked up in an abyss of thick darkness. Whereas others in such a situation may discern a ray of light in the thick cloud of darkness, the depressed individual sees nothing but darkness, darkness, darkness.

TREATMENT OF ANXIETY AND DEPRESSION

Come unto me, all ye that labour and are heavy laden, and I will give you rest. Take my yoke upon you, and learn of me; for I am meek and lowly in heart: and ye shall find rest unto your souls. For my yoke is easy, and my burden is light. Mathew 11:28-30

Be careful for nothing; but in everything by prayer and supplication with thanksgiving let your requests be made known unto God. Philippians 4:6

Before I look at the possibilities at the disposal of medical care to treat depression I would like to make an observation.

Anxiety that leads to depression is brought about, among other things, by cares, worries, poverty, marital problems, disease, job loss, etc. I am not saying these are pleasant moments for anyone to go through. Indeed, I wish sincerely, from the bottom of my heart, that Almighty God would spare all of us trials of any kind.

Since, as I have stressed all along, we live in a fallen world, there is no guarantee, however, that we shall always be spared trouble. How do we react in such a situation?

As Christians, there is no other place to run to but to Christ our Lord. Indeed, we must cultivate an attitude of looking up to Christ in all situations, whether good or bad.

> *Be careful for nothing; but in everything by prayer and supplication with thanksgiving let your requests be made known unto God. Philippians 4:6*

This does not imply, however, that we are not to do all that is within our means to solve the problems that come our way. Indeed, one of my favourite sayings is, "God helps those who help themselves." Indeed, we have to work to provide for the needs of ourselves and our family, to preserve our property, etc.

We are, however, called upon to develop a strong confidence in Almighty God, the trust and confidence that will free our minds from anxiety. We are called upon to cultivate a sense of dependence on His provisions, the sense of dependence on Him that will keep us calm and stable no matter the circumstances.

Our circumstances, like the weather, the weather of the British Isles, can change at short notice. By the same token, our joyful circumstances today may change tomorrow. The stability of work can change at any moment. If we look to circumstances rather than Christ we could well end up like Peter who, as he walked on the waves at the command of the Lord, turned to look at the storm, yes, the circumstances and then began all of a sudden to sink!

DRUG TREATMENT OF ANXIETY AND DEPRESSION

While not denying the fact that medication can have a favourable influence in mental illnesses such as anxiety, panic disorders, depression etc., it is my conviction that when it comes to diseases of the mind, the effect of medication, in many instances, is inadequate.

Let us take depression as an example. You may have read or heard that the condition is caused by a chemical imbalance in the brain. The chemical imbalance theory revolves around a chemical known as serotonin. According to this theory, low levels of serotonin in the brain lead to depression. All that is needed according to this school of thought is to give the patient medication that will correct the chemical balance, yes, cause an increase in serotonin in the brain of the patient and hurray, the patient will once again be happy, happy, happy!

Following this thinking, a group of medication, the selective serotonin re-uptake inhibitors or SSRIs, was introduced in the therapy of depression.

Selective serotonin re-uptake inhibitor, as its name implies, has the goal of preventing the re-absorption of serotonin from the brain back into the bloodstream. With an increase in the concentration of serotonin in the brain, it is hoped that the patient will feel better again.

This obviously does not tell the whole story. Now we know that in several instances of patients suffering from depression, the individuals involved were living a normal life, free from depression, before an acute life event set in to cause their malaise.

Let us take the example of a married couple who are enjoying a harmonious and fulfilling marriage, who are in fact so happy they appear to be swimming in heavenly bliss. In the midst of their happiness, tragedy strikes—one of them dies through tragic circumstances. The other is thrown into severe depression which lingers on for several months. Now, how does brain chemistry, indeed, how does the shortage of serotonin in the brain explain this kind of depression? Carrying the argument further, how can medication, which has the sole effect of increasing the concentration of serotonin in the brain, help such an individual?

Depression indeed is a complex medical condition. Several factors come into play to bring it about. In the same way, we should not rely only on medication for a cure. As far as Christians are concerned, in my opinion, emphasis should be placed on Bible-based counselling backed by prayer and, where possible, fasting.

Having said that, I shall now list some of the anti-depressants in use:

- Selective serotonin re-uptake inhibitors (SSRIs): I have already touched on these. An example of this group of medication is Citalopram.
- Atypical antidepressants: These are described as atypical antidepressants because medical science does not understand exactly the mechanisms of their action. An example is Mirtazapine.
- Tricyclic antidepressants (TCAs): An example of this group is amitriptyline.
- Monoamine oxidase inhibitors (MAOIs): An example is Phenelzine (Nardil)

The antidepressants listed above have one thing in common: they all have considerable side effects—side effects that could be so severe as to lead to the interruption of therapy.

Plant-based drugs: Apart from the above-named group of medication, a few plant-based drugs are used in the treatment of anxiety and depression. An example is St. John's wort (*Hypericum perforatum*) which is popular, especially in Germany.

NON-DRUG THERAPY

Apart from medication, *psychotherapy* is employed in the treatment of anxiety and depression. One may want to know what the term stands for.

It is a branch of psychiatry which employs dialogue and a variety of communication techniques with the aim of treating individuals suffering from mental and emotional disorders. In the treatment of depression, psychotherapy aims at helping the patient develop new ways to cope with challenges in life, and to identify and understand more about depression and how to avoid it in the future.

Psychotherapy is also known as "talk" therapy. During the talking sessions that may take place in groups or on a one-to-one basis, the skilled psychotherapist may use one or more of the following strategies:

- Pinpoint the life problems that contributed to the patient's depression, and help him or her to understand which aspects of those problems he or she may be able to solve or improve.
- Identify negative or distorted thinking patterns that contribute to feelings of hopelessness and helplessness that accompany depression.
- Explore other learned thoughts and behaviours that create problems and contribute to depression.
- Help people regain a sense of control and pleasure in life.

Much as these measures in this type of therapy may help an individual in the short run, as far as I am concerned, in the long run, it is only the freedom that we have in Christ that will free us from the burdens that may come our way as a result of our fallen nature.

Christians should, in my opinion, aim at Bible-based counselling by spirit filled pastors and other co-workers in the church. As I mentioned earlier, in all such cases we should back our effort with prayer and if possible fasting.

Chapter 34

Good Night And Sleep Well

∞

INSOMNIA

Insomnia is the chronic inability to fall asleep or remain asleep for an adequate length of time.

The brain requires regular and adequate sleep to regenerate itself so that it may continue to function properly. This inevitably leads to the question: how much sleep is adequate for the human being? A new-born usually sleeps between 16 and 19 hours per day; this reduces to about 12 hours by the age of 5 years. For most adults, 7 to 8 hours a night appears to be the best amount of sleep, although the amount ranges from 5 hours to 10 hours of sleep each day depending on the individual.

Unfortunately in the modern world, due to various reasons—domestic and work demands, social responsibilities, unhealthy lifestyles (some sit before the computer and play games deep, deep into the night!)—it is becoming increasingly difficult for some individuals to get adequate sleep.

ON THE USE OF SLEEPING TABLETS

For those who suffer from chronic sleeplessness, sleeping tablets can be an answer. It is important, though, that therapy aims first at the root cause of the problem rather than the symptoms. Lack of sleep could be secondary to depression which in turn could be a result of burdens on the mind that need to be alleviated.

After several weeks of use, sleeping pills begin to lose their efficacy, which may call for an increase in dosage to achieve the desired effect. In the end one could become addicted to them.

Before you consider buying over-the-counter sleeping tablets or asking your doctor to prescribe those requiring a doctor's prescription, you may consider the following tips aimed at promoting a more restful and effective sleep:

- It is important to have a good bedtime routine. As far as possible try to go to bed at about the same time every night. This should be the case whether one is tired or not.
- The bedroom should have the right environment, not too hot or cold; not too noisy.
- One should undertake some moderate exercise every day— swimming, walking or jogging. This is particularly important for people who have a sedentary lifestyle or who are not engaged in strenuous physical work.
- It is important to avoid any stimulant drinks, especially coffee several hours before the fall of darkness.
- One should also avoid eating too much late into the night.
- Some have reported that drinking a cup or two of milk or chamomile tea before retiring to bed has a favourable influence on sleep.
- Listening to music, restful gospel music, is also reported to help induce sleep.

Good night and sleep well, dear reader!

www.ingramcontent.com/pod-product-compliance
Lightning Source LLC
Chambersburg PA
CBHW030009290326
41934CB00005B/270